How to
control
wrinkles
and
ageing

How to
control wrinkles
and ageing

Parvesh Handa

NEW DAWN PRESS, INC.
USA• UK• INDIA

NEW DAWN PRESS GROUP

Published by New Dawn Press Group
New Dawn Press, Inc., 244 South Randall Rd # 90, Elgin, IL 60123
e-mail: sales@newdawnpress.com

New Dawn Press, 2 Tintern Close, Slough, Berkshire, SL1-2TB, UK
e-mail: sterlingdis@yahoo.co.uk

New Dawn Press (An Imprint of Sterling Publishers (P) Ltd.)
A-59, Okhla Industrial Area, Phase-II, New Delhi-110020
e-mail: sterlingpublishers@airtelmail.in
www.sterlingpublishers.com

How to Control Wrinkles and Ageing
Copyright © 2006 Parvesh Handa
ISBN 978-1-84557-607-3
Reprint 2007, 2008

PRINTED IN INDIA

CONTENTS

CHAPTER–1

KNOW
YOUR BODY

Ageing is the process of growing old and is marked by signs of changes in the external appearance as well as internal functioning of the human body. However, contrary to common perception, the ageing process is not inevitable or irreversible.

To look young and feel fit with the passage of time, there is a need to achieve self-grooming. For arresting the negative effects of ageing, it is essential to have a thorough knowledge of the working of the human body and its major systems and explore its specific structures (anatomy) and functions (physiology). The major body systems are Integumentory System, Skeletal System, Muscular System, Respiratory System, Circulatory System, Digestive System, Genito-Urinary System, Nervous System and Endocrine System.

The Cells

The human organism is made of a vast variety of parts that vary in complexity. These include organ systems, individual organs, tissues and cells. The cell is the basic structure from which all other body structures are made. The human body is composed entirely of cells, fluid and cellular products.

Cells are made up of protoplasm, a colourless, jelly-like substance in which food elements such as protein, fats, carbohydrates, mineral salts and water are present.

As long as the cell receives an adequate supply of food, oxygen and water, it eliminates waste products and continues to grow and thrive. In case these conditions do not exist and there is the presence of toxins, the growth and the health of the cells are impaired. When the cell reaches maturity, reproduction takes place by direct (amitosis) or indirect (mitosis) division. The indirect method of reproduction occurs in human tissues.

Metabolism

It is a complex chemical process whereby the body cells are nourished and supplied with energy to carry on their activities. Metabolism is the series of chemical reactions which utilise nutrients for growth, repair or energy production within the body. It is the rate at which the body uses energy for the process of metabolism. The energy is measured in kilocalories (kcal) or kilo joules. One calorie is the amount of energy required to raise the temperature of 1 kg of water by 1°C. Joule is the metric unit of measurement for heat and energy (1kcal : 4.2 kj). The table below shows energy value of nutrients:

Nutrient	Energy value/g
Carbohydrates	3.75 k cal (16 kj)
Protein	4.00 Cal (17 kj)
Fat	9.00 Cal (37 kj)

Energy requirements

The amount of food a person requires depends on the energy used each day. This varies according to the age, sex, body structure, occupation, physical activities, and conditions such as pregnancy or ill health. In fact, ideally the food eaten each day should supply no more and no less than the amount of energy used that day. The average energy requirements for an adult woman is approx. 1940 k cal and for a man 2550 k cal. Occupations are classified according to how active they are, as follows:

Sedentary:　　　Office worker, teacher, shop worker

Moderate active: Hairdresser, beauty therapist, postman

Very active:　　Construction labourer, athlete, hockey/ football player

Special needs:　Extra energy is required during the final months of pregnancy and breast feeding

Basal Metabolic Rate (BMR)

This is the amount of energy required to keep the body alive when it is warm and at complete rest. It is used to keep the heart, lungs and the digestive system working to maintain brain, functioning of body and all the chemical reactions in the body. Women tend to have a lower BMR than men because they are lighter and have less muscle tissue. BMR is also lower in elderly people and during periods of starvation, when the body needs lower food energy.

The average values for BMR for a person aged 40 years are:

Women:　1360 kcal (5700 kj) per day

Men:　　1750 kcal (7300 kj) per day

Table below illustrates the energy used for various activities for an average female (25-year-old office worker weighing 62 kg):

Activity	K Cal/hour	kj/hour
Sleeping	57	238
Sitting (eating)	66	300
Standing (cooking)	126	540
Washing and dressing	126	540
Washing at moderate pace	210	900
Walking up/down stairs	390	1680
Office sitting	90	360
Office walking	156	660
Dancing	270	1140
Average jogging	390	1620

In case of the following conditions, seek advice of a doctor, before following the suggestions in this book:

- Age under 18 or over 70 years
- Undergoing medical treatments
- Severe obesity
- On a medically prescribed diet
- Pregnancy or feeding a child

There are two phases of metabolism: *anabolism* and *catabolism*. Anabolism is a process of building up larger molecules from smaller ones and catabolism is the breaking down of larger substances or molecules into smaller ones and hence releasing energy. Both anabolism and catabolism are carried out simultaneously and continuously in the cells so that their activities such as energy releasing reactions are balanced with energy consuming reactions. However, if we use less energy than we manufacture, we may notice a weight gain. To get rid of built-up fat, more energy must be used or less energy (through food) taken in.

The body is made up of millions of individual tiny microscopic cells which are built into tissues, organs, and glands. *Body tissues* are composed of groups of cells and are of five types i.e., Connective tissue, Muscular tissue, Nerve tissue, Epithelial tissue and Liquid tissue which carries food, waste products and hormones by means of the blood and lymph.

Organs are structures designed to accomplish a definite function. The most important organs of the body are: the brain (which controls the body), the heart (which circulates the blood), the lungs (which supply oxygen to the blood and control respiratory system in the body), the liver (which removes toxic products), the kidneys (which 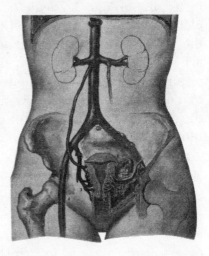 excrete waste products), the stomach and intestines (which digest the food).

The Skeletal System

Personal appearance is determined by general body structure which depends on the skeleton. The skeletal system which is the physical foundation or framework of human body, is composed of different shaped bones, cartilages and ligaments united by movable and immovable joints which vary from person to person according to race, sex and age. The skeleton is divided into three main regions such as the skull, the spine and the limbs. In the skull, several bones unite together to protect the brain. The skull rotates on the spine and the position of the skull is adjustable to aid the senses of seeing, smelling and hearing. The brain controls the whole body and mental stability. The *Spine* is made up of many irregular shaped bones having elastic tissues which permit flexibility. The spinal column keeps the body and head erect. Ribs circle around the body from the spine and meet in front at the breast bone. The ribs aid in respiration and hold the heart and lungs and control blood pressure. *Respiration* is the controlled exchange of the gases—oxygen and carbon dioxide by the cells to activate the energy. The blood carries oxygen from the respiratory system and nutrients from the digestive system to the cells where they are absorbed in five different ways: diffusion, osmosis, dissolution, active transport and filtration.

The blood pressure increases during emotion, excitement and anger. It lowers during sleep and rest depending upon age, sex, mental exertion and physical work of the individual. Too much physical exertion, keeping late nights, excessive use of alcohol, consuming excessive salt and habit of irregularity in taking food are harmful. *Bone* is the hardest structure in the body and is found in several forms such as flat bones (The Skull), long bones (legs and arms) and irregular bones (spine). Bones have several functions in the body such as to give shape and strength to the body, to protect organs from injury, to serve as an attachment for muscles and to control bodily movements. The point of junction of two or more bones is called a joint.

Common conditions affecting skeletal system are spondylitis, arthritis (inflammation of joints), bunion (swelling of joint), bursitis (inflamed knees), gout (pain in the joints), kyphosis (concave curve of the spine), Lordosis (convex curve of spine), osteomyclitis (inflammation of the bones), and slipped disc.

Respiratory System

Respiratory system is situated within the chest cavity protected by the ribs. The diaphragm is a muscular partition that separates the chest from the abdominal region and controls breathing. The main input, vital to maintaining life is oxygen. Using this oxygen, the body produces carbon dioxide which is released from the body when we breathe out. This process is known as respiration. Remember, oxygen is more essential than either food or water. A man may live for 60 days without food, a few days without water but if deprived of oxygen, he will die in a few minutes. Nasal breathing is healthier than mouth breathing because the air is warmed by the surface capillaries, and the bacteria in the air are caught by the hairs that line the mucous membrane of the nasal passages. The rate of breathing depends on the individual's activity and energy expenditure, which increase the body's demand for oxygen; as a result the rate of breathing is increased. A man needs about three times more oxygen when walking than when standing. Lungs are spongy tissues composed of microscopic cells that take in air. These tiny air cells are enclosed in a skin-like tissue. During inhalation, oxygen is absorbed into the blood. The cycle of breathing and exchange of gases is repeated many thousands of times in a day and is vital to the life of every individual cell, tissue, organ and system of the body. The respiratory system can be divided into two main groups:

- Upper respiratory tract which consists of nose (nasal and turbinate bones), sinuses (air space in nasal bones), pharynx (nasal cavity which leads to back of the throat) and larynx (passageway which leads to upper throat)
- Lower respiratory tract which consists of trachea (windpipe), bronchi (passageway to both lungs) and lungs (soft, spongy tissues on either side of the heart

within thorax). The lower respiratory tract consists of 12 pairs of ribs, 12 thoracic vertebrae and the sternum.

Breathing (the movement of air in and out of lungs)

Inspiration (breathing in):
- Diaphragm contracts pushing abdominal cavity down
- Intercostal muscles contract
- Ribs are pulled up and out
- Thoracic cavity enlarges
- The pressure in the lungs decreases
- The pressure of the incoming air increases
- Air rushes into the lungs.
- Lungs expand as they fill with air.

Expiration (breathing out):
- Diaphragm relaxes and returns to dome shape.
- Ribs return to normal position.
- Thoracic cavity returns to original shape.
- The pressure in the lungs increases.
- The pressure of the air outside decreases.
- The air is able to flow out of lungs.
- Elastic recoil of lungs helps to force air out
- Contraction of the abdominal muscles will aid forced expiration

Common conditions affecting the respiratory system include asthma (difficulty in breathing), bronchitis (inflammation of the lining of the bronchi), common cold (contagious viral infection), croup (viral infection that affects children) also known as barking cough, emphysema (inflammation in the lungs generally in old age), grandular fever (viral infection most common in the 15 to 22 year age group), hayfever (an allergy to pollen which affects the nose, eyes and sinuses), hyper-ventilation (rapid deep breathing), laryngitis (loss of voice), lung cancer (tumour in the lungs), pharyngitis (inflammation of the pharnyx), pneumonia (viral infection causing chest pain, dry cough, fever etc.), pleurisy (inflammation of the pleurs surrounding the lungs), pnemothorax (collapsed lung), rhinitis (causing blocked, runny and stuffy nose) and tuberculosis (infectious disease in lungs)

Circulatory System

Circulatory or vascular system is vitally related to the maintenance of good health. This system controls the steady circulation of blood through the body by means of the heart and blood vessels such as the arteries, veins and capillaries. The blood-vascular system consists of heart and blood vessels for the circulation of blood. Another division—the lymphatic system consists of lymph glands and vessels through which the lymph circulates. Both the systems are linked with each other.

Blood circulation is a two-way system – transporting substances such as oxygen, water and nutrients necessary for the body and transporting unwanted substances such as carbon dioxide and waste products away from the body. The system functions as follows:

- Oxygen enters the lungs as we inhale.
- Blood picks up oxygen in the lungs.
- Blood carries oxygen to the heart.
- Heart pumps blood to the cells.
- Blood vessels carry oxygen to the cells.
- Oxygen is given to the cells.
- Cells give carbon dioxide to the blood.
- Blood vessels carry carbon dioxide to the heart.
- Heart pumps carbon dioxide to the lungs.

- The circle completes when the carbon dioxide leaves the lungs as we exhale.

The Heart

It is a muscular, conical-shaped organ located in the chest cavity, and is enclosed in a membrane. The heart is made up of three layers of tissues – endocardium or inner layer forming the lining of the heart, myocardium or middle layer made up of cardiac tissues which control producing contraction in the form of heartbeat and pericardium or outer layer forming a double layer. The space between the layers is filled with a fluid to prevent friction. At the normal resting rate, the heart beats about 72 to 80 times in a minute. The heart beats approximately 130 times per minute in a new born baby. The heart is divided into four sections by four valves.

The Blood

It is the nutritive fluid circulating through the circulatory system. It is sticky, salty fluid with a normal temperature of 98.6 degree Fahrenheit (37 degree Celsius) which makes up about one-twentieth of the weight of the body. Blood is bright red in colour in arteries and dark in veins. The change of colour is due to the exchange of carbon dioxide for oxygen as the blood circulates throughout the body.

The primary functions of the blood are:

- It carries water, oxygen, food and secretions to all cells of the body.
- It carries away carbon dioxide and waste products to be eliminated through the lungs, skin, kidneys and large intestines.
- It helps to stabilise the body temperature, thus protecting the body from extreme heat and cold.

- It aids in protecting the body from harmful bacteria and infections.
- It clots the blood, thereby closing injured minute blood vessels and preventing the loss of blood.

There are three main types of blood cells: erythrocytes or red blood cells (which have a life of about 120 days and are removed from the body by the liver or the spleen; these contain haemoglobin (haemo=iron and globin=protein) that contribute the red colour of the blood), leucocytes or white blood cells (these colourless cells have a life span between just a few hours and few years depending upon their activities) and thromobocytes or platelets (fragile cells which have a life span of 5-9 days).

Lymphatic system (The Lymph-vascular system)

The lymphatic system acts as an aid to the blood system. Lymph is a colourless, watery fluid that carries on an interchange with the blood, carries nourishment from the blood to the body cells, acts as defense against invading bacteria and toxins, removes waste material from the body cells to the blood and provides a suitable fluid environment for the cells.

Blood pressure

It is the pumping action of the heart caused by relaxation and contraction of the ventricles. The maximum pressure associated with the contraction of the ventricles is systolic pressure whereas the minimum pressure associated with the relaxation of the ventricles is diastolic pressure. The normal blood pressure in an adult is approximately 120 systolic over 80 diastolic and is maintained by the force of the heartbeat. High blood pressure (hypertension) occurs when the heart has to work harder to force the blood.

Common conditions affecting the circulatory system include anaemia (a decrease in the production of haemoglobin), angina (reduction of blood supply to the heart by excessive exertion), aneurysm (swelling of an artery), arteritis (inflammation of an artery), coronary thrombosis (a common cause of heart attacks), diabetes (whereby the body cannot use the sugar and carbohydrates from the diet), heart failure (heart weakness), haemorrhoid (varicose veins in the rectum or anus, also known as piles), hepatitis B or C (inflammation of the liver due to viruses transmitted by infected blood), leukaemia (over-production of white blood cells resulting in blood cancer), rheumatic fever (inflammation of heart which often follows tonsillitis), septicaemia (blood poisoning) and thrombus (a blood clot in the blood vessel or the heart).

Muscular System

The human body comprises more than 500 muscles which contribute 40 to 50 percent of the total body weight. They are contractible, elastic, fibrous tissue which produce movement of every part of the body. Each muscle contains its own nerve and blood supply. Striated muscles (those having lines and furrows) include facial, arms and leg muscles while non-striated muscles function in the stomach and intestines. The cardiac muscle is the heart itself. Muscles need nutrients and oxygen which are supplied by the blood. Regular exercise strengthens body muscles and prevents formation of extra fat at various regions of the body— usually around the stomach, waistline, trunk, hips, back muscles, abdomen and the neck.

Common disorders of muscular system include cramp (painful contraction of muscle), fatigue (build-up of lactic acid in muscle), fibrosiris (inflammation of muscle fibres), muscular dystrophies (collapse of muscle), myasthenia gravis (weak muscles), myonoma (a tumour composed of muscular tissue), myotonia (muscular contraction), paralysis (muscle failure), rupture (tearing of muscle), spasm (sudden muscle contraction), strain (overuse of muscles), stress (muscular tension), tendinitis (inflammation of muscle) and torticollis (contraction of neck muscles). To look after muscular system, drink water before, during and after exercise as well as at regular intervals throughout the day. Have nutritious food containing carbohydrates, proteins and vitamins. Adequate rest and a balance of varied activity play an important part in maintaining healthy muscles.

Digestive System

Digestion is the process of converting food into a form that can be assimilated by the body. The digestive process starts in the mouth and is completed in the intestine passing through pharynx, food pipe and the stomach, the complete process taking about nine hours. The digestive system is assisted by organs such as the gall bladder, pancreas and liver. Common conditions which affect the digestive system are anorexia (a psychological eating disorder), bulimia (associated with over-eating), colitis (inflammation of the large intestine), constipation (infrequent, dry passing of waste), diarrhoea (frequent elimination of faeces), dehydration (weakness due to loss of nutrients from the body), dysentery (infection of the large intestine), flatulence (air in the stomach), gastro-enteritis (inflammation of the stomach and intestines), proctitis (inflammation of the lining of the rectum), ulcers (over production of acid).

The efficient functioning of the digestive system ensures that the cells, tissues, organs and systems of the body are provided with the nutrients and water necessary for survival. The body loses about 1.5 litres of water a day through the kidneys (as urine), through the lungs (as breathing out), and sweat (through the skin). The body makes about a third of a litre of water a day through energy production in the body cells. The food we eat can be classified as carbohydrates, proteins, fats, vitamins, minerals and insoluble fibre. The following measures are to be taken to maintain fluid balance in the body and ensure adequate nutrition to provide sufficient energy and sustain activity.

- Drink sufficient quantity of water to avoid dehydration.
- Take fresh, unprocessed food for maximum nutritional value.
- Avoid intense activity during and after eating.
- Eat when hungry, not out of habit. Avoid indigestion.
- Maintain efficient, regular elimination.
- Chew food well to assist the mechanical digestion.
- Avoid stress.
- Avoid fried food contributing to premature ageing.
- Avoid intense emotional excitement and fatigue.

The Reproductive System

Female reproductive system includes the ovaries, the fallopian tubes, the uterus and the vagina. The functions of this system are the production of hormones and reproduction. The reproductive organs are different in a male and female although their prime functions are similar. The testes in males and ovaries in females are known as sex glands and are responsible for producing male and female sex hormones respectively. The testes produce male hormones known as androgens which include testosterone and the ovaries are responsible for producing female hormones, estrogen and progesterone. In males, these hormones are responsible for producing the sexual characteristics associated with puberty which include development of sperm, the change of voice and growth of facial hair etc. In females, they are responsible for the onset of the menstrual cycle, development of breasts and eventually the menopause. The onset of puberty equips a male and female to produce a new human being. Reproduction is a process which ends in a female during the menopause when the ovaries stop developing new ovum every month although a male of the same age is still capable of producing healthy sperm.

Reproduction begins with fertilisation. Semen from the male is introduced into the female during sexual intercourse. The sperms present in the semen travel into the uterus and the fallopian tubes. If an ovum is present, the sperm penetrates it so that fertilisation can take place. The nucleus of the sperm fuses with the nucleus of ovum to form an embryo. This process of reproduction belongs to a category known as mitosis. An embryo is formed which develops further in the uterus until it becomes a foetus and finally into a child in a process which takes approximately 40 weeks.

The Endocrine System

It acts as the main communication centre of the human body. It consists of a set of endocrine glands, each gland responsible for the production of hormones. A hormone is a chemical substance which has the ability to effect changes in other cells. It is secreted directly into the blood stream and transported to various systems of the body. Hormones are produced from the components of food we eat—either protein based or fat based. The main—endocrine glands includes one pituitary gland (located at the base of brain), one tiny pineal gland (located in the brain), one thyroid gland (located in the neck), four parathyroid glands (located on the sides of the thyroid glands in the neck), one thymus gland (located in the thorax), two adrenal glands (located on the top of each kidney), two ovaries located in the lower abdomen in women and two testes (located in the groin in men).

The secretion of hormones is controlled by the hypothalamus, the nervous system and internal environment of the body. These are excreted from the body in urine. Hormone imbalance takes place when the endocrine glands produce either too much or too little of the hormones which results in malfunction of organs. Sex hormones are responsible for the development of breasts, the menstrual cycle, the reproductive organs becoming functional, hair growth (in underarm and pubic area) in women, production of sperm and semen, the breaking of the voice, increased growth of muscles and bones and hair growth on the face, pubic area, underarm, abdomen and chest in men: A female body goes through various stages of sexual development which include puberty, menstrual cycle, pregnancy and menopause. Puberty marks the onset of sexual development when ovaries in females and testes in males are stimulated into activity by the production of sex hormones. Every month the uterus in a female is prepared for the fertilisation of an egg. The menstrual cycle is usually approximately 28 days. Pregnancy occurs when fertilisation is successful; the placenta develops during pregnancy, which forms a direct link between the foetus and its mother. Menopause marks the end of child bearing years in women and usually starts between the age of the 45-55 when the hormone level changes and the menstrual cycle becomes irregular and eventually stops altogether. The other symptoms include short-term flushing, sweating, loss of bone mass, loss of pubic and under arm hair and thinning of skin.

Female Disorders

Amenorrhoea
Cancer
Cervical Erosion
Ecotopic Pregnancy

Endometrosis

Thrush

Urethora

Addison Disease

Fibroids

Galactorrtoea

Hirsutism

Polycystic Ovarian Syndrome

Pre-menstrual Syndrome

Virilism

Disorders for Male and Female

Cystistis

Prostitis

Sexual Transmitted Disease

Acromegaly

Conn's Syndrome

Dwarfism

Common disorders affecting the genito-urinary, nervous and endocrine systems in women include – amenorrhoea (absence/stoppage of menses), cervical erosion (at the neck of womb with a slight discharge), cystitis (frequent urge to pass urine), ectopic pregnancy (when fertilised ovum develops outside of the uterus usually in fallopian tube), endometriosis (cells from the uterus formed in fallopian tubes or ovaries), thrush (infection of vagina causing itchiness and discharge), urethritis (inflammation of the urethra), acromegaly (over-secretion of the growth hormone in pituitary gland), Addison disease (disorder of adrenal glands causing muscular weakness, irregular menstrual cycle and dehydration), fibroids (development of non-cancerous tumours in the uterus), galactorrhoea (excessive milk flow caused by over secretion in the anterior pituitary gland), hirsutism (over production of testosterone in females loading to unwanted hair growth), Polycystic Ovarian Syndrome (irregular menstrual cycle and sometimes infertility), Pre-menstrual Syndrome (swollen, tender breast, mood swings etc.), virilism (increased body and facial hair and deepening of voice in women). Prostatitis (inflammation of the prostate gland), gynaecomastia (over production of oestrogen in males causing the development of breast), cancer (developing in breast, ovaries, bladder and uterus), Sexually transmitted diseases (acquired through sexual contact), Conn's syndrome (over-secretion of aldosterone usually causing high blood pressure and kidney failure), dwarfism (under-secretion of hormones from anterior pituitary gland resulting in failure of the growth in bones and organs) are other diseases of the endocrine system.

Integumentory System

It plays an important role in the human body as it consists of the skin, hair and nails which provide the body with a water-proof protective covering. The skin consists of layers of fatty tissue. The outermost layer of skin is called the epidermis, beneath which lies the dermis and finally the hypodermis. Hair follicles on the skin and scalp are tube-like structures within which a hair develops and grows through a pore—a minute opening in the skin surface. Each follicle has a rich blood supply feeding the cells. Sebaceous glands are generally attached to the hair follicles and produce skin's natural lubricant—an oily substance called sebum. Nails do not have a growth cycle like hair and grow approximately 4 cm per year. The prominent conditions affecting the skin and hair include Abscess, Acne Vulgaris, Skin Allergy, Alopecia (Baldness in patches on the scalp), Boil, Cellulitis, Herpes simplex, Dandruff (Pityriasis capitis), Dermatitis (Eczema), Moles, Psoriasis,

Papule, Ringworm, Scabies, Seborrhoea, Pustules, Skin Tags, Stretch marks, Hirsutism (superfluous hair), Urticaria and Vitiligo. The basic factors for addressing the disorders of skin, hair and nails are :-

1. Ingestion of adequate quantity of water.

2. Intake of essential natural antioxidants (Vitamin A, C and E).

3. Rich balanced diet.

4. Rest (Minimum 6-8 hours sleep every day allows the body and skin to replenish and regenerate).

5. Physical activity to stimulate the circulation ensuring skin an active blood supply.

Skin

Know Your Skin

The skin is usually of five types : normal, dry, greasy, mixed and sensitive. The skin is the largest organ of the body with a surface area of 1.62 sq. meters in average adult male and 1.43 sq. meter in an adult female. It consists of three components – the epidermis, the dermis and the hypodermis.

Epidermis

The outermost layer (the layer you can feel and see) has a thickness between 0.07 and 0.12 mm (0.08 to 1.4 mm on sole of the feet and palms of hands). The epidermis consists of five layers. Skin cells are formed in the innermost layer (the basal cell layer or stratum germinativum) and push their way to the outermost layer (the horny layer of stratum corneum). In the process, the live cells change into dead, hard, flattened cells. Dead cells on the surface are constantly being shed or rubbed off, making way for newer cells from below. The horny layers in the epidermis is the body's layer of defence. The horny layer prevents most substances from diffusing into lower layers, only very light oils and identical substances can penetrate deeper. The basal cell layer also produces primarily flattened cells called keratinocytes and melanocytes which produce a substance called melanin. Melanocytes are stimulated to produce melanin by the ultraviolet (UV) rays in sunlight. Melanin is a dark pigment which blocks UV rays. The greater the exposure to sunlight, the greater the production of melanin. The epidermis has three principal functions such as protecting the body from the environment (particularly the sun), preventing excessive water loss from the body and protecting the body from infection.

Dermis

It is the foundation of the skin. It contains blood and lymphatic vessels, sweat glands, hair follicles, sebaceous glands and nerve endings. These are held together by collagen and elastin fibres, which together give skin its strength and flexibility. Blood and lymphatic vessels in the skin bring nutrients to skin cells and carry away wastes. They also act as heat regulators. When you feel hot, these vessels dilate and carry more fluid, radiating heat to the outside. When you feel cold, they contract, reducing the flow of fluid to the body's surface to preserve body heat. Sweat glands also help regulate temperature by producing sweat which evaporates from the surface to lower skin temperatures. Hair follicles produce hair. The sebaceous glands produce sebum. An excess of sebum makes skin look and feel oily. The functions of the dermis include:

- Rendering mechanical protection to the body from bumps and knocks.
- Providing oxygen and nutrients to the body via blood in vessels.
- Removing waste products of metabolism from epidermis.

- Providing shape and form to the body by holding all structures.

- Contributing to skin colour.

- Regulation of body temperature through blood and sweating.

- Skin sensations of touch, pain, heat and cold.

The dermis is also the biggest storehouse of a substance called sterol which in itself is of no use to the body. It is, however, converted into Vitamin D by the action of ultra violet rays in sunlight, hence a certain amount of sunlight is good for the body.

Subcutaneous Layer
It is a fatty region that is not considered part of the skin.

Composition of Skin
The whole skin is made up of cells. One square inch of skin consists of 19,500,00 cells which include 19,500 sensory cells, 65 muscles, 78 nerves, 1300 nerve endings, 13 sensory nerves for cold, 78 sensory nerves for heat, 95 sebaceous glands, 630 sweat glands and 20 blood vessels. Nerves are of three types i.e. *motor nerves* (distributed to the blood vessels), *sensory nerves* (which react the heat, cold, touch, pressure and pain) and *secretory nerves* (distributed to oil and sweat glands). The glands in this part of the body are of two types – *sebaceous gland* (secreting oil and found in large number on the face, back and scalp) and *pseudoferous gland* (secreting salt water, urea and other waste products on to the skin).

Functions of the Skin
- Acts as covering for the body to protect from heat, cold, bacteria, harmful elements and environment conditions.

- Regulates the temperature of the body. It secretes sweat in case of extreme heat.

- Breathes in oxygen and takes out unwanted gases.
- Eliminates salt and waste products in the form of sweat.
- Secretes sebum (a type of oil) which keeps the skin smooth and soft.
- Holds moisture which keeps the skin soft and moist.
- Nerve endings make us aware of sensations like heat, cold, pressure and pain.

Skin Diseases

Blemishes

The human body has been given a most beautiful covering – the skin. Nothing is more lovely and attractive for a glowing healthy skin. Skin may not appear to be as vital an organ as the heart or a brain, but nevertheless presence of intact skin is essential for life. Skin disease can make life unbearable. Skin is the first line of defence against the germs that might enter the body. Enzymes on the surface of the skin destroy germs, provided the skin is healthy and intact. But small breaks and tears in the surface of the skin may open the way to infection in the deeper tissues as well. Skin disorders are of various kinds, but few of them are very harmful causing premature ageing:

Allergy

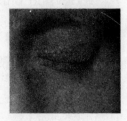

It is a sensitivity caused by contact with certain types of food, cosmetics, medicine, tints etc., which may result in itching and inflammation accompanied by redness, swelling, blisters, oozing and sealing.

Acne and Pimples

Acne Vulgaris is a common inflammatory disease of the skin mostly affecting the face and the upper part of the chest and back caused by seborrhoea and hormonal disturbances usually during adolescence. Acne is more common and severe in boys than girls. Never break the pustules or squeeze it, else they will become septic and leave permanent scars. The predisposing factors e.g., 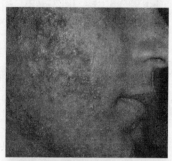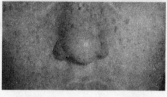 disorder of digestive tract, hypovitaminosis of Vitamin A, E and B, anaemic condition, malnutrition, infection, the character of diet and metabolism, overeating and excessive use of cosmetics and hereditary influences are some of the causes of this disorder.

Scabies

Scabies is a contagious disease caused by a mite. This mite lays eggs in the burrows in the skin. The disease spreads through contact with infected individual, 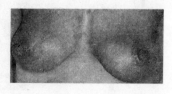 clothings, bedding and the commonly affected parts are finger webs, palm, wrist, front of arms, soles, areas around the breast, nipples and genitals. The sole complaint is severe itching which is more at night. The infection due to mite may cause small papules.

Eczema (Dermatitis)

An inflammatory skin disorder in which a cuticle is fissured with a sticky, watery discharge. It starts with redness due to dilated blood vessels. Fluid accumulates in the skin scabs and crusts. Apply paste of *babchi* mixed with mustard oil or leaves of *mahua* (Indian Butter Tree) smeared with sesame oil on the affected skin.

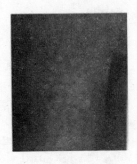

Fungal Infections

Common fungal infections are ringworm and candidiasis. Ringworm is a patch on the body especially between the legs, on the face, the neck, the back and on the buttocks. It is also known as *tinea corporis*. It is caused by inflammatory infection of the skin produced by certain moulds. Scratch the affected skin and apply borax mixed to lime juice. Apply marigold juice or leaves of basil on infection.

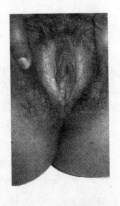

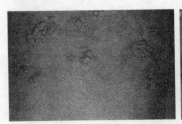
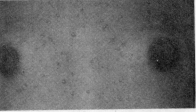

Candidiasis is caused by *candida albicans*. It is common in patients who have a fancy for taking antibiotic drug or use of oral contraceptives. It may involve skin, intestines and vagina (Vulva Vaginitis).

Freckles, Moles and Warts

Freckles are small flat, irregular brownish spots on the skin often due to exposure to sun. Mix a tablespoon of milk cream to few drops of lime juice and apply at night. Grind turmeric and sesame seed to make a paste and apply on the affected skin.

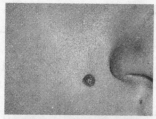

Warts are pink, brown and black swellings usually by a defect of the melanocytes which multiply and grow down into the dermis. They are excised by electro-surgery or surgical

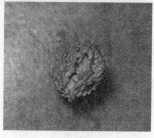

diathermy. Warts are also seen in different forms on the soles of feet and in the genital and rectal areas due to virus infection.

Boils and Carbuncles

A boil is a tender swelling in the skin surrounded by a large red area. A carbuncle is a group of boils close together, which may later form one very large boil. Boils are painful in areas where the skin is closely attached to the underlying tissues, such as on the nose, ears or fingers.

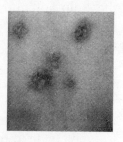

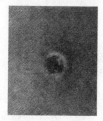

Apply warm moist compresses three to four times a day over the tender area to help easy drainage of boil. Area of surrounding skin should be bathed with neem soap to kill germs and avoid further spread of the infection.

Psoriasis and Vitiligo

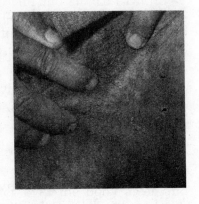

Psoriasis (*eka kusha*) is a scaly eruption of the skin in which red patches develop covered by scale which can be itchy. It is caused due to impurities in the blood associated with emotional factors. Neem leaves ground and applied on the affected area will be helpful.

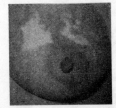

Vitiligo are the white patches of the skin caused by destruction of melanocytes caused mostly due to hormonal imbalance.

Seborrhoeic Dermatitis

A chronic inflammation of the skin most frequently seen on the scalp. Inflammation may begin on the skin behind the ears and later on the scalp, then to the eyebrows, fold of nose and breasts.

Types of Skin

There are six types of skin:

1. *Normal Skin* : It has the characteristics of unblemished velvety texture, having a clear appearance, an even colour, feels neither tight nor greasy, soft and supple to touch and a high degree of elasticity. Failure to look after the normal skin or abuse by sun, wind or cold leads to dry and damaged skin leaving it prone to premature development of lines and wrinkles.

2. *Dry Skin* : It has the characteristics of feeling tight, stretchy and irritable. It often looks flaky, develops fine

lines and wrinkles around the eyes, tightens and becomes rough or scaly after washing with soap. The skin is stretched after prolonged exposure to low humidity. If neglected, dry skin looks cracked, has reduced production of sebum and becomes rough or scaly.

3. *Oily Skin* : It is also called seborhoeic skin. It generally appears at puberty (it starts earlier from the age of six upwards in few cases). However, the problem is rare after the age of 35. Usually, it involves only the upper part of the body, where sebaceous glands are found in excess. This type of skin is common in adolescents and young adults due to increase in sebum production under influence of the male sex hormones. After washing, the skin becomes glossy and moist.

4. *Mixed Skin* : It is also called combination skin, which has dry and oily patches. It is characterised on the face by thickened, shiny skin with patches of dry skin.

5. *Sensitive Skin* : It is easily irritated. Most people with this condition are allergic to contact with cosmetic products. It is more common among women and amount of sensitivity varies from skin to skin. The cheeks become red veined or sore and chapped in cold weather.

6. *Matured Skin* : It shows the characteristics of dry skin. Looks very parched, saggy and dehydrated if no skin care has been practised during younger age. The matured skin is deeply lined and loose due to lack of moisture.

Skin Care

If you are below 15 : The skin is usually clear, smooth and youthful. The application of cosmetics should be avoided except for a moisturising cream in cold weather and a sun barrier cream while venturing out in the hot sun. Skin cleansing assists in clearing blackheads in adolescence.

If you are between 16 to 20 : The only essential is a moisturiser especially when the skin is dry and has blemishes. However, a light tinted cream or liquid foundation can be used to add colour if the skin is pale. A cleanser is essential before going to bed.

If you are between 21 to 30: A good routine followed in this age pays handsome dividends later on in 30s and 40s. Plenty of cleanser and moisturiser are essential. If the skin is normal and dry, use moisturiser and in case of oily skin a light easily absorbed skin tonic or astringent should be applied.

If you are between 30 to 40 : During these years the first fine lines appear. A richer skin tonic at night protects from cold or hot weather. Moisturiser also helps considerably.

If you are between 40 to 55 : Lines and wrinkles settle more firmly unless the skin is nourished with rich lubricating creams and moisturising agents. Facials help to keep skin in good condition, using a rich face mask followed by a moisturiser and light skin tonic is recommended.

If you are 55 and above : Avoid soap and too hot or too cold water. No hard massaging over the body. Skin firming preparations help to retain the contours of the face and the body.

Cleansing, moisturising and toning are the important steps in caring for the skin.

Cleansing : It is the first step while caring for the skin by removing perspiration, grease, dust, stale make-up, dirt and bacteria before retiring to bed. Pay particular attention to the creases of nose, under chin area, neck and ear lobes with a light upward and outward movement. The cleansing cream should be kept on the skin for at least 30 seconds.

Toning : Hormone creams and lotions, vitamin products, serum ampules, anti-wrinkle creams and lotions come in the nourishing group of skin-care products and give the skin youthful appearance. Skin toning removes greasiness, closes skin pores, freshens the skin and leaves a smooth clean texture, holds the foundation and powder for long and stimulates the blood supply.

Moisturising : All skin types need moisturiser – even the oily types. But for a dry skin a moisturiser is vital. Moisturiser is applied after cleansing and toning and always before applying make-up. Nourishing creams which are skin tonics relax tight muscles and accelerate circulation.

Astringent : It is used to tone the skin and remove last traces of grease and closes pores.

Lines and Wrinkles in Early Age ?

The sun, rain, wind, heat, cold, and all natural phenomena can have an adverse effect on the skin, hence skin care should be adapted to changes in climate. Wrinkles, blackheads, pimples, acne vulgaris, skin inflammations, dermatitis, eczema, ringworm, freckles and scabies are chronic skin disorders and allergies which mar lovely faces. Cleaning, moisturising, nourishing, toning the skin are essential processes to avoid these skin disorders. The warning symptoms when care should be taken is the stage the skin becomes over dry as the sebaceous glands become less active. When skin loses its elasticity, wrinkles appear due to the cross linking and hardening of collagen fibres. Other warning symptoms are when epidermis of the skin appears thinner, the broken capillaries appear on the cheeks and around the nose, the facial contours become slack reducing the muscle tone, the blood circulation becomes poor leaving the skin appearing sallow, patches of pigmentation appear on skin's surface and dark circles and puffiness occur under the eyes.

Skin Care throughout Life :

- *Infant skin* : Premature babies oftenly have very little subcutaneous fat resulting in their skin lying loosely over their muscles and bones. The skin of premature baby can comprise up to 13% of its body weight, compared with 3% in an adult. Lubricants such as creams, emollients and baby lotions or oil may be used for newborn babies, to prevent or treat dryness of the skin. Methods of prevention of chapping and nappy rashes include keeping the skin dry with frequent nappy changes. Barrier products also remove harmful skin bacteria and help in reducing diaper dermatitis.

- *Childhood Skin* : It shows little or no damage from sunlight. The care of the skin of small children is almost entirely in the hands of parents. The skin does not need moisturising unless there is atopy or eczema or after prolonged exposure to sun or sea.

- *Teenage Skin* : It is the time of life at which the body starts to produce greatly increased amounts of sex hormones. Both girls and boys produce male hormones called androgens. Under the influence of these androgens the skin produces more grease (sebum) and in most teenagers there is a tendency for spots to develop—anything from simple blackheads to large pustules. Caring for teenage skin is a matter of balancing the cleansing and toning needed to remove the excess grease with adequate moisturising to combat the over drying effects.

- *Adult Skin* : Our skin changes inexorably as we get older. A young adult's skin is well-hydrated, tends to be soft, smooth and supple, and has a natural translucency. A mature adult skin tends to function less well. Ultimately it may become dry and tend to feel tight, with a rough texture and dull appearance and wrinkles start to appear.

- *Mature Skin :* As women get older their skin matures, and particularly after menopause declining oestrogen may lead to dehydration of the stratum corneum which tends to make the skin look thinner and older than it really is. For cleansing, it may be advisable to use soap-free cleansers for the body. For use on the facial skin, it is essential to choose a suitable moisturising cream which gives sufficient protection against dehydration.

- *Elderly Skin :* By the time an individual becomes a senior citizen, the skin may well have experienced decades of sun exposure associated with the effects of intrinsic ageing. Elderly skin can be very dry and almost paper thin. Such type of skin becomes more fragile and prone to injuries, broken veins, small blood vessels becoming vulnerable to burst. Day and night moisturisers help combat the decline in skin function. It is still important to continue protecting the skin against the sun.

How Skin Changes with Age : A Summary

Age (yrs)	Appearance	Physiology
Upto 15	Smooth texture skin	Good skin hydration
15-25	Acne Key factor	High sebaceous gland activity
25-45	Appearance of wrinkles & sagging	Drop in skin hydration
45-55	Rough texture, more wrinkles	Thinning of epidermis, dry skin
55 +	Wrinkles, fine lines, sagging	Low production of collagen, over–production of melanin

CHAPTER–2

FACIALS AND FACE PACKS TO REJUVENATE SKIN

Do you have a soft, smooth, clear, attractive and glowing skin on your face? If so, you are blessed with a priceless gift and are the fortunate one. But mind you, the beauty of your skin will not last long. With advancing age, there is no guarantee that you will maintain that fresh youthful look. You will have to exert to keep it as it is. Normally, worries and tensions, coupled with the climatic effect, tell upon the skin and many women look aged even in their prime. Facial routines keep up your youthful glow, and it is advisable to look after your skin on a regular basis. To have a natural beauty is a blessing but most people tend to lose it through their own negligence. As soon as a female reaches adolescence, she is attracted towards artificial cosmetics. The excessive use of make-up makes one lose her natural beauty. The pores of the skin get clogged by these cosmetics preventing the carbon dioxide inside our body from coming out and also preventing fresh oxygen entering the body. This results in the skin losing its original glow and regaining lost beauty is extremely difficult. Facials keep the face attractive, maintaining soft texture and sheen.

Facials

Facial treatments are divided into two categories such as:

Preservative

Those aimed at maintaining the health of facial skin by correct cleaning methods, increased circulation, relaxation of the nerves and activation of the skin glands and metabolism through massage come under this category.

Corrective

Those aimed at correcting facial skin conditions such as dryness, oiliness, blackheads, ageing, lines and minor conditions of acne come under this category. The nine stages of facials include:

Stage 1 : Cleansing is done with cleaning milk, cream and lotion. Cleansing is more important than massage as it deep cleanses the skin and clears up the pores. Cleansing is done in three steps as follows.

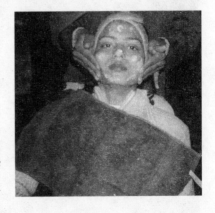

- Take a small piece of cotton, moisten it in plain water and spread cleansing cream. Hold the cotton in both hands and start cleansing face.

- Remove 'bindi' in clockwise, anti-clockwise and criss-cross direction.

- Then remove lipstick starting from lower lip. Take another piece of cotton and remove eye make-up. To cleanse make-up, crisscross above the chin and under the lips. Start from chin to jaw line to the temple then from lip line high up to the temple, then below the

eyes. Now clean upper lip, sides of the nose, bridge of
the nose, tip of the nose, sides of the nose up to the
temple, clean forehead with zig-zag stroke and meet at
the temple point. Now clean jaw and neck in crisscross
strokes, clean the shoulder clockwise, anti-clockwise.
Clean the shoulder blade, sides of the neck and meet
behind the ear. Take a fresh piece of moist cotton and
remove all the cleaning cream on the face.

Stage 2 : Manual Massage (15-20 minutes). Massage is given
with massage cream, chilled water is to be used in summer

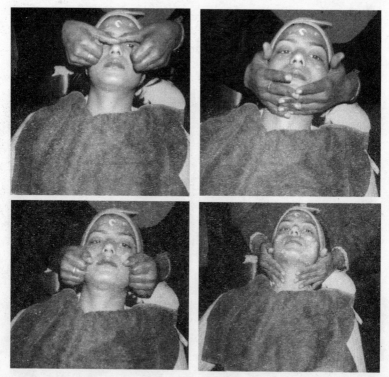

and tap water in winter. Add little raw milk (1/2 cup) in
three cups of water to cut down the consumption of the
cream. Massage is divided into five parts – general stroke,
eye massage, forehead, jaw line and neck and sternum

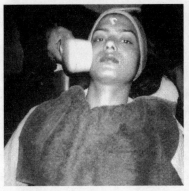 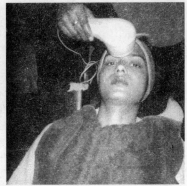

Stage 3 : Vibratory massage (5-7 minutes) is given with an electrical gadget called vibratory massager. Never give massage on bare skin. Do direct massaging on the cheeks and shoulder, indirect massage is given on the eyes. Never give massage on the lips.

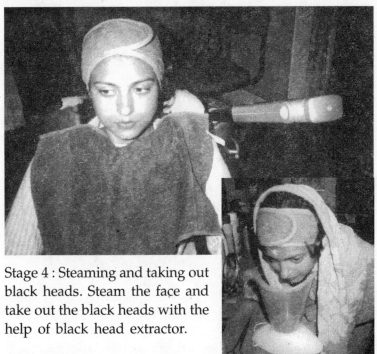

Stage 4 : Steaming and taking out black heads. Steam the face and take out the black heads with the help of black head extractor.

Stage 5 : Cold Compression – Dip the cotton in chilled water adding rose water to it. Always use chilled water in summer and tap water in winter.

Stage 6 : Application of mask or face pack (25-30 minutes) : Apply face pack according to the type of skin. While removing pack give mild rubbing with light hand. Never give harsh treatment to the skin.

Stage 7 : Ultra Sonic Oxilation (30-40 minutes) – It is a mild steam given to the skin to provide deep moisture.

Stage 8 : Cryo waves is given to the skin by means of chilled waves or sprays. It helps to close down the pores and protects skin from getting dehydrated. It improves the blood circulation and helps in settling down the skin.

Stage 9 : Sun protection – Apply sun protection cream or lotion.

Facial: Why and How Often ?

Facial is beneficial for cleansing the skin, increasing circulation, activating glandular activity, relaxing nerves, maintaining muscle tone, strengthening weak muscle tissue, correcting skin disorders, preventing formation of lines and wrinkles on the face, softening and improving skin texture and complexion, giving a youthful feeling and adding to the confidence. Facial is one of the most restful treatments that offers relaxation, stimulation and soothing effects and enhances application of an attractive make-up. Facial can be given as often as once a week, once in a fortnight and once a month according to the requirement. The following precautions must be taken while doing facial :

- Ensure relaxed and quiet atmosphere and maintain neat and clean sanitary conditions.
- Analyse skin before facial treatment. Remove make-up to determine : If the skin is dry or oily? If black heads or acne are present ? If broken capillaries are visible ?

If the texture of the skin is soft or velvety or harsh and rough ?. This analysis will determine the choice of creams and face packs to be used in massage movements, the amount of pressure to be applied while massaging, the type of make-up to be applied after facial treatment and the areas on the face that need extra attention.

- Feel relaxed while doing facial and perform all work as noiselessly as possible.

- Follow systemic procedure such as, in case your hands are cold, warm them before starting facial treatment, keep your nails smooth so as not to scratch the skin while doing facial.

- Remove neck and ear jewellery before starting facial and place the same in purse. Remove dress and hang it up. Remove shoes. Place towel near the facial bed or chair. Protect the hair by fastening a headband around hair. Adjust clean towel from shoulders draping across chest and across middle of back.

- Do not dip your fingers into a preparation. All packs and creams should be removed from their containers with a spatula.

- For giving a facial you need equipment, implements and materials such as cleansing lotion or cream, emollient cream, astringent lotion, antiseptic solution, talcum powder, witch hazel, cleansing tissues, absorbent cotton, cotton pad, headband, towels, tray, clean sheet or drape, facial steamer, infra-red lamp and lanolin or hormones cream for dry skin.

Don'ts When Giving a Facial

- Don't give a facial if you suffer from offensive body. Odour or tobacco smell or foul breath.
- Don't give excessive or rough massage.

- Don't have rough nails.
- Don't use too hot towel or steam the face for too long.
- Don't use infra-red lamp for more than five minutes.
- Don't be careless of sanitary requirements.
- Don't use substandard facial creams or other substances.
- Don't be in the habit of talking too much or being tense while getting facial manipulations.
- Don't be careless in removing cream behind the ears or under the chin or in other areas on the face.

Procedure for a Simple Facial

1. *Cleansing routine* : Remove make-up from the face (including lipstick). Apply cream over the face using both hands—start from chin, lift the chin, slide fingers to temples, rotate with pressure upwards, slide to left eyebrow, then stroke up to hairline gradually moving hands across forehead to right eyebrow. Take additional cream and blend. In long even strokes, smooth down the neck, chest and back. These are optional manipulations. Start massage at the forehead, lightly around the eyes, temples and back to forehead. Slide down nose to upper lip, glide to temples and forehead, cover lightly to chin, then firmly up jaw line, again to temples and forehead. Remove cleansing cream with tissues or warm moist towel. Start at forehead and follow the contours. Remove all cream from the face and finish with neck and back.

2. *Steaming the face* : Steam face mildly with warm moist towel or facial steamer and remove blackheads. Sponge face with antiseptic.

3. *Massage techniques* : Apply emollient (tissue) cream to face, neck, shoulders and chest. Apply eye cream around the eyes and muscle oil around the neck. Massage the

face; give manipulations using the hands (slightly cupped) and fingers. Start under the lower lip, press outwards in a continuous line with two fingers. Repeat several times. Pinch gently along the jaw line, working outwards. Press along the entire hair-line, working towards ears.

4. *Optional manipulations*: Have manipulations (optional) over chest, back and neck areas before starting the regular facial. Apply massage cream, give manipulations using rotary and circular movements. Use rotary movement across chest and shoulders, to spine, then to base of neck, ear and earlobe in circular movement. Rotate six times, then remove cream with tissues or warm moist towel. Dust the back lightly with talcum powder and smooth.

5. *Important pressure points on the body*: There are several reflex points on the face, pressing these point help to improve the circulation and energy flow in the face and also tone the skin. Hold each point for five seconds. These points are situated on the face, hands and feet, and other parts of the body.

   • If the face looks tired or is sagging, rub at the centre of lower cheekbone or at the outer corners of eyes on both sides of the face.

   • In case of puffy eyes, rub on either side of the nose.

   • In case of droopy cheeks/jowls, rub the hollows just below the ears.

   • In case of eye bags and loose cheek muscles, rub the border line between eye socket and cheekbone on both sides of the face.

   • To tone up and energise the muscles of the entire body, rub at the centre of the palms of both hands.

The Important Facial Massage Movements

Massage movements are usually directed towards the origin of a muscle with the middle and ring fingers over the delicate skin of upper lip, eyes, nose and forehead, which bruise easily.

1. *Linear movement* : Apply with fingers rotating with upward stroke, usually on forehead and temples.

2. *Circular movement* : Start at eyebrow line towards the hairline over forehead.

3. *Criss-cross movement* : Start at side of forehead and back.

4. *Stroking movement* : Slide fingers over brows on forehead and move towards temples.

5. *Brow and eye movement* : Place middle fingers at inner corners of eyes and index fingers over brows. Slide towards outer corners of eyes, under eyes and back to inner corners.

6. *Nose and upper cheek movement* : Slide fingers across the cheeks and temples.

7. *Mouth and nose movement* : Apply circular movement on the mouth, sides of nose and brows.

8. *Lip and chin movement* : From centre of upper lip, towards lower lip and chin.

9. *Optional movements* : Draw fingers under lower lip, centre of upper lip around the mouth.

10. *Lifting movement of cheeks* : From nose to ears on cheeks.

11. *Rotary movement* : Massage from chin, mouth and nose to ears on the cheeks.

12. *Light tapping movement* : Working from chin, mouth, nose to ear and across forehead.

13. *Stroking movement* : Applying light upward strokes over the neck, in front, side and downward with pressure.

14. *Circular movement* : Starting at back of ears, apply circular movement over shoulders and across the chest.

Do you have dry skin?

Insufficient flow of sebum from the sebaceous glands makes skin dry. For more effective results, expose face and neck to infra-red lamp upto 5 minutes. Avoid using lotions which contain alcohol. Apply skin lotion suitable for dry skin. Apply eye cream over and under the eye and lubricating oil over the neck.

Procedure for facial for dry skin with high-frequency current

Give manipulations using indirect high-frequency current for not more than 5 minutes. Sponge the face and the neck with skin freshener, then apply a moisturiser.

If your skin is oily?

An oily skin is prone to blackheads. Apply cleansing lotion and remove with moist cotton pads or sponges. Steam the face to open the pores and press out blackheads. Sponge the face with astringent. Apply massage cream, give manipulations and remove the cream. Now apply astringent lotion to the face to close the pores. Blot excess moisture with tissues.

If you have acne skin?

Clean the face. Apply acne cream or ointment all over the face and neck. Use high-frequency current over the affected skin for not over five minutes. Remove acne cream with tissues. Apply a pack suitable for acne skin for ten minutes, Remove the mask and blot with a wet towel. Steam face and extract blackheads. Apply astringent lotion. Avoid use of make-up on an acne skin.

How to do 30-minute home facial?

It is the quickest way to revive and liven up jaded skin. Cleanse face and neck with cleansing milk. Apply cream all over the face and blend it thoroughly, massaging face and neck in an upward direction. Apply a face-pack. Lie on the back and apply face mask on for 15 to 20 minutes till it dries. When it is dry, wash face and neck with cold water. Dry the skin and apply moisturiser.

Is your skin prone to wrinkles?

Hot oil mask facial is very beneficial for dry, scaly skin prone to wrinkles.

Give a plain facial. Moisten facial gauze with warm oil and place on the face, to hold mask ingredients that do not cling or hold together on the face.

Apply infra-red rays for 5 to 10 minutes. Remove the mask and apply moisturising cream.

Remove cream with a warm, moist towel and apply astringent lotion followed by moisturiser.

Do you have sensitive and dehydrated skin?

Vitamin C facial is very useful for sensitive and dehydrated skin.

- Cleanse with cream, milk or lotion.
- Massage with friction.
- Lymphatic and normal massage manipulations (10 - 15 minutes).
- Apply peeling facial mask.
- Vitamin C fluid on face.
- Venus massage followed by High Frequency treatment.

If you have a post acne skin?

Oxygen bath facial treatment is most suited for young, mature and post acne skin. Sometimes, after facial treatment 2-3 acne appear on the face, which is a good sign. Procedure for oxygen bath facial treatment is as follows:

- Cleansing the skin with cream, milk or lotion.
- Steam the face for opening skin pores (3 to 5 minutes).
- Apply vitamin cream on oily skin. In case of dry skin, mint gel should be applied with normal massage (10 to 15 minutes).
- Application of oxygen rich mask heals acne. High frequency treatment (for 4-5 minutes) is recommended.

If you have ageing, wrinkled skin?

Thermoherby pack facial is useful for ageing, wrinkled, dry skin.

- Cleanse with cream, milk or lotion.
- Massage for 15-30 minutes.
- Apply thermo herb pack.
- Remove blackheads followed by cold compression.

Alfa hydroxy acid treatment facial

It consists of the following steps :

- Cleansing.
- Suction (with softening milk).
- Steaming the face with friction massage. Application of cream.
- Lymphatic massage.
- Removal of blackheads.
- High frequency current for less than five minutes to remove infection.

- Application of protein mask (20-minutes) for acne or oily skin.

Vegetable peeling facial

It is useful for oily skin without pimple and acne. It has the following steps.

- Cleansing with rose water.
- High frequency or ozone treatment.
- Application of vegetable peel pack when semi-dry.
- Application of medicated cream. Leave it for 5-7 minutes. Apply fruit/vegetable juice (preferably cucumber juice or raw milk).
- Removal of black heads.
- Cold compression followed by application of sun protection cream.

European Facial Techniques

It includes step by step procedures and routines for an extensive facial massage, hand massage, hot towel wrap after application of masks. Sponges are used to clean make-up thoroughly and applying creams and moisturisers. Steamer is used and exfoliation is done.

Express Facial (25 minutes)

This facial routine comprises combination of relaxation, cleansing, warm compresses, soothing massage and nourishing herbal extracts which leaves the skin revitalised and moisturised.

Classic Facial (50 minutes)

This facial is a great way to begin the balancing process for the skin. The facial includes deep pore cleansing, exfoliation to remove dull surface skin cells, gentle extraction to remove deeper impurities and a mask that will benefit your exact skin type and specific needs.

Anti-ageing Facial (50 minutes)

It is a unique combination of powerful antioxidants and nourishing essential oils which leave delicate skin velvety, smooth and supple. This facial is ideal for sensitive or environmentally stressed skin types.

Hydraderm Facial

It is a high-tech skin therapy which makes use of mild electrical currents that deeply cleanse, hydrate, regenerate and oxygenate skin, and result in excellent treatment leading to visible improvement immediately with long-lasting effect.

Hydradermine Lightening Facial

It is a beauty treatment with visible, lasting results, promoting fresh skin. In this facial active lightening ingredients are diffused by gentle ionisation to procure a radiant, clear, visibly lighter and even complexion.

Faritas Evidence Facial

It is an anti-ageing treatment which adds minerals, moisturises the skin and restores facial firmness.

Super Hydraderm Facial

This stimulating facial uses specific eye and neck products. Throughout the facial intensive movements are used to improve elastic hydration for eyes and neck. The result for this treatment is immediate and long-lasting.

Faritas Aromaplasty Facial

Rich in protein and vitamins, this treatment is to rebalance and harmonise the skin. Aromatherapy oils are used to remove impurities and to revitalise and stimulate the skin.

Reflexology and Relaxation (Therapeutic Massages) Facial

A 75-minute treatment in which finger pressure is applied to the reflex zone of the feet to stimulate the internal organs and systems of the body, helping to activate the body's natural healing ability and to restore balance. Afterward a relaxing massage promotes further release of tension in the nervous and muscular systems, resulting in a deep state of relaxation and rest.

Reflexology in the neck and head

A 30-minute treatment focused on the zones of the head and neck produces a decongestive effect, stimulates blood circulation, reduces inflammation, lowers blood pressure and is ideal for migraine and headache. Highly relaxing and strongly recommended for eliminating stress.

Relaxing Massage

A special, 50-minute treatment for relieving accumulated stress, reducing muscle fatigue, and improving blood circulation.

Sports Massage

A 50-minute treatment before or after sports activities. Helps to maximize performance potential, reduces muscle fatigue and eliminates toxins produced in the muscles during physical exercise.

Therapeutic Massage

Ideal for treatment of sensitive areas affected by muscular tension, stress and fatigue.

Anti-Cellulite Massage

A reductive massage that works on zones with the highest concentrations of cellulite. Special movements are used to generate heat to help dissolve body fat. Ideally, it should be followed with a sauna session and completed with a shower treatment.

Lymphatic Drainage

The massage therapy technique that helps to detoxify the skin and promote its renewal. Helps to drain toxins and prevent premature ageing.

Thai Massage

Traditional Thai massage is a combination of acupressure, breathing techniques, gentle stretches and beautiful postures. Thai massage stimulates the free flow of energy along the lines and balance is restored to the whole – physically, emotionally, mentally and spiritually leaving one relaxed and revitalized, reducing stress and relieving soft tissue pain.

The roots of Thai massage are in India and arrived in Thailand around the same time as Buddhism in 3rd century B.C. Indian doctor Jivaka Kumar, Baccha, a physician is regarded as 'Father of Thai massage in India. Thai massage, ideally performed on a mattress on the floor has several benefits as follows:

- Provides muscular and general relaxation.
- Helps in stress reduction, pain management, recovery from injury, health promotion, circulation of blood and lymph and restoration of metabolic balance.
- Releases points of tension in the body which block the natural flow of energy.
- Releases strength, increases energy and flexibility leaving deep relaxation, pressure on feet and legs.
- Assists alignment and postural integrity of the body.
- Strengthens the internal organs of body, thus promotes inner peace.
- Suitable for post-natal care and improving neurological functions.

A traditional Thai massage takes every joint through its full range of movement and stretch of every muscle, leaving body fully relaxed and revitalised.

Shiatsu Massage

It is an oriental massage in which the fingers, palms and sometimes elbows are used to exercise pressure on specific points of the body to stimulate energy channels and the internal organs. Reduces stress, alleviates aches, pains, fatigue, and the symptoms of a variety of diseases.

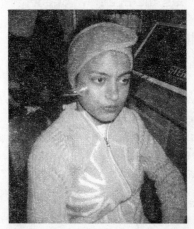 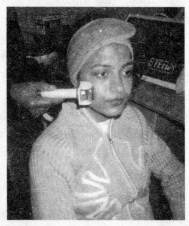

Ultra Sonic Massage Therapy

Provides glow, improves blood circulation, activates sebaceous glands, improves dry skin and is especially effective for dull and sallow skin. It works through an electric device and is a highly effective massage treatment in deep penetration of skin ideal to perform in winter.

Suction Massage Therapy

This massage therapy can suck out infection, unfriendly bacteria, dirt, dust, germs from the deeper stratum of the upper layer of the epidermis. This electric therapy which is performed by the compressor is totally safe. The benefits include tightening of skin and it leaves skin germs-free, helps in controlling sebum, improves blood circulation and removes infections.

Ozone Therapy

This includes using Alkaline rays for both scalp and facial skin treatments (such as itchy scalp, dandruff, acne, pimples) This therapy is performed using anti-allergic, antiseptic and sterlised powder.

Micro Therapy

It is a power massaging therapy to treat ageing skins, showing signs of laugh lines, frown lines, crow's feet. This therapy helps improve blood circulation, stimulate nerves and muscles, regenerate cells and tissues, and promote the elastic fibres of the skin to assist in face- lifting.

H.F. Therapy

The primary action of this treatment is thermal heat producing due to rapid vibration but without muscular contractions. This therapy helps in solving eye disorders and contributes life-long physiotherapy techniques to give instant and excellent results. The beneficial result of HF therapy include relieving dark circles, puffiness under eyes and treatment of crow's feet and shrunken eyes.

Dermabrasion

Various skin problems are solved by this therapy in which layer of the skin damaged due to acne, scars, blemishes and pigmentation marks causing uneven tone, is removed. The various benefits include levelling the surface of skin, reducing scars and solving tanning.

Aroma therapy facial

An aroma therapy facial consists of steps such as cleansing, use of natural refreshing tonic, herbal compress, essential oil massage, application of compress or poultice, facial mask, application of moisturisers and finally rest. The facial routine is similar to nine stage simple facial. Custom-design the face mask. A pack should always be applied after applying a scrubber, because scrubber opens the pore and it becomes necessary to close down the pores with the help of face pack. Pack is left on the face for 10 to 15 minutes, then washed off. If the skin is very wrinkled or very dry, then the mask should be removed when it is semi-dry. Face packs are of the following types :

For normal skin

Make a paste of two tablespoons of gram flour and four tablespoons of milk and apply all over the face and neck for ten minutes.

For oily skin

Make a paste of two tablespoons of honey with one teaspoon of lemon juice and one teaspoon of rose water, apply all over the face for five minutes.

For dry skin

Use a pack of one tablespoon milk powder with one teaspoon of gram flour and two tablespoons of rose water on for 15 to 20 minutes.

For tanned skin

Mix a teaspoon of curd ten ground almonds. Use the pack to remove tan and soften the skin.

For dull skin

Mix *multani mitti,* brewer's yeast and rose water. Apply to the face for 15 minutes to nourish the skin.

For pimply skin

Rub a piece of sandalwood on a clean stone using a little rose water or cucumber juice. Apply paste on the face to feel a tingling fresh feeling.

For blemished skin

Make a paste of gram flour, kaolin, fuller's earth and dry milk powder. This face pack tightens the skin pores.

Antiseptic pack

Make a paste of crushed neem leaves with toner or astringent for curing pimples, acne and scarred skin.

Oil control pack

Mix orange juice with astringent and apply on the face with cotton on oily skin.

Skin tightening pack

For dull, wrinkled skin beat an egg and mix to it rose water or toner.

Cleansing pack

Grind cucumber (peeled) and mix to it rose water. Good for all types of skins.

Ayurvedic Packs for Skin

We are born with, soft and smooth skin, but most women cannot maintain the same texture and tone even during teens. Like any other living tissue, skin too responds to tender care and attention. Ayurveda – the spiritual health science gives traditional herbal rejuvenative ways to maintain youth and correct imbalance of body and mind. *Doshas* to the skin are identified as *Vatta* (Dry), *Pitta* (Sensitive) and *Kapha* (Oily). Modern herbal treatments for different skin needs are given here:

Vatta: (Dry) To prepare the pack, collect one teaspoon each of almond powder, dry milk, *ashwagandha* powder and sugar. Make a fine paste with rose water or sandal water or milk. Apply a thick layer on body skin, dry for 15-20 minutes, then wash with plenty of water. Another body pack is prepared by mixing pulp of two ripe bananas with mashed water melon and 1/2 teaspoon honey and glycerine. Apply thick paste on body, wait to dry, then wash.

Pitta (Sensitive): Mix 1 teaspoon each of orange peel and *manjistha* with ½ teaspoon each of *daruhaldi* and neem. Add to it neem or *triphala* water and apply the paste on the body till it dries. Another pack is prepared by mixing 1/2 teaspoon each of *dhania* powder and *manjishtha* and 1 teaspoon each of *chandan* powder and *trifla* powder with honey or coconut water or cucumber water. In case of blemishes on the skin, apply a paste mixing apple, cabbage, grapes and tomato.

Kapha (Oily): Mix 1 teaspoon each of barley (peel) and lemon (peel) with half teaspoon each of orange (peel) and *lodhra*. Add to it neem or mint water to make a paste, apply and allow to dry. Do not scrub, wash or remove with water. Another pack is prepared by mixing 2 teaspoons salamli with ¼ teaspoon alum powder and fresh aloe vera gel. Apply for 15-20 minutes and wash when it dries. The third type of pack can be prepared by mixing 1 cup fresh pineapple with ½ cup fresh papaya and 2 teaspoons honey. Apply pack to the full body. Allow to dry for 30 minutes and take a bath afterwards.

Gadgets Used in Facials

Suction : An electrically operated gadget which sucks out the infection from the upper layer of epidermis and from the deeper layers by cosmetic products (cleansing milk or vitamin used milk or softening milk).

Brushing : An electronic gadget which helps in removing dirt, impurities, grease and dead cells from the skin during facial treatment. The pumice stone having corrosive action helps in peeling of dead cells from the skin.

Vapozone (Facial steamer) : An electrically operated gadget which produces a moist, uniform heat to produce steam and cleanse the skin. It warms the skin, cleans skin pores and induces the flow of blood, oil and sweat. Vapozone can also be used for cold, spraying rose water over the face with control.

CHAPTER–3

BODY MASSAGE TECHNIQUES

Massage is one of the oldest and most useful natural methods of physical treatment. It is performed by means of the hands or with the aid of mechanical or electrical appliances: such as therapeutic lamps, high frequency facial steamers and vibra-massagers to certain areas of the body, mainly the face, neck, shoulders, the upper chest, back, hands, arms and the scalp and when done properly, the skin becomes flexible and attractive. To master the technique, a through knowledge of anatomy of the body and considerable practice in performing the various movements is required. Hands doing the massaging should be kept soft by the use of creams, oils and lotions to prevent damage to the tissues. The nails should be short and smooth to prevent any scratching on skin. The wrist and the fingers should be flexible and the palms firm, warm and dry. Massage should not be done on persons having a weak heart, high blood pressure, inflamed and swollen joints, glandular swelling, abrasion of the skin, broken capillaries of the skin and skin diseases. Massage improves, develops and tones up the muscular tissues, beautifies the skin and preserves its suppleness. By the action of the hands and fingers, organic waste products can be driven into the blood stream and eliminated. Progressive massage gives the body a chance to free itself from toxic matter, and gain elegance and good health. Massage should be done preferably in the morning, after the toilet routine. If you do not have time in the morning, massage at night before going to bed. It should last for 20 to 30 minutes and each area should be massaged for two to five minutes covering the neck, the arms, the legs, the shoulders, the neck, the back, the buttocks, the hips and abdomen. For slimming massage and anti-cellulitis, use appropriate cream available in the market. Massaging with oil once a week makes the skin supple. End the massage by taking an alternately hot and cold shower and a friction rub with a coarse towel or wash cloth. Wrinkles are the first sign of ageing and are an alarming signal. Whether you have lumpy, flabby, withered or sallow skin and wrinkles on the skin, your face can regain the appearance of youth under the action of your fingers. Regular daily massage prevents wrinkles on the forehead, temples, eyes, nose, cheeks, mouth and chin.

Do's and Don'ts:

To ensure good results here are a few suggestions.

1. Protect your hair with a bandeau and wash your hands.

2. Cosmetics clog the skin pores. Remove all make-up.

3. If skin is oily, use complexion milk with pH acid. If skin is dry, use cleansing milk with witch hazel base. If skin is dehydrated, use a moisturising lotion to avoid herpes and wrinkles. If skin is too moist, use an astringent lotion to clear pale and puffy look.

4. Apply vitamin cream to your face before starting a massage.

5. Use a slimming cream, if your facial features have a tendency to plumpness.

6. Cotton seed oil is most commonly used for massaging but butter is used for filling out cheeks, the neck and also for breast enlargement.

7. Oil should not be used for persons with excessive body hair. The oil should be washed off completely after massage.

8. Body massage may be done for 40-45 minutes. It is however, not recommended in serious inflammatory cases of the joints and infectious diseases which cause formation of pus which may spread to the entire system. In these cases, affected part should first be bathed with hot water for 15 to 30 minutes, then massage should be done for a few minutes.

9. Avoid deep pressure on swollen nerves, for it will increase the inflammation.

10. Sleeplessness can be cured by slow and gentle massage on spine and back.

11. Abdominal massage is beneficial in constipation. It stimulates and tones up the abdominal muscles. Abdominal massage should not be done in case of hernia, inflammation of the uterus, bladder, ovaries and fallopian tubes, kidney stones, ulcers of the stomach and intestines, and pregnancy. Avoid abdominal massage after heavy meal. The bladder should be emptied before the massage. Persons with hypertension should also avoid abdominal massage.

12. Chest massage strengthens the chest muscles, increases circulation and tones up the nervous system of the chest, heart and lungs.

13. Massage of back stimulates the nerves and circulation and is used for treating backache, rheumatic afflictions of the back muscles and for soothing the nervous system.

Basic Massage Manipulations

The basic movements are *stroking* (effleurage), *kneading* (petrissage), *friction* (deep rubbing), *percussion* (tapotement) and *vibrating* (shaking). Massage movements are basically of two types depending on the desired effect—relaxing and toning. Relaxing movements are slow and soothing whereas toning movements are rapid and energetic. Stroking movements consist of running hand very lightly with palms of the hands and pads of the fingers upwards, never downwards. They are frequently applied to the forehead, face, scalp, back, shoulders, neck, chest, arms and hands. Kneading movements help to clear waste matter from the muscles, activate the nutrition of the tissues, remove fatigue and increase nervous and muscular energy. They consist of light but firm and deeper movement. This movement is beneficial for the chin and the cheeks. Friction movement is employed with fingers and palms on face and neck. In percussion movement, stimulation is done briskly with the finger tips. This increases blood supply, soothes nerves and strengthens muscles. Vibrating movement is achieved by rapidly shaking, vibrating and pressing. Use hands or fingers on the body in vibrating movement to increase glandular activity and stimulate nervous plexuses.

Physiological Effects

To obtain proper results from a scalp or facial massage, one must have a thorough knowledge of all the structure involved—the muscles, the nerves and the blood vessels all of which have pressure points. A skilful massage positively influences the structure and function of the body by activating the circulation, secretion, nutrition and excretion of the skin. The frequency of massage depends upon the age and condition to be treated but in general a weekly massage is recommended. A facial and scalp massage nourishes the skin and its structures, reduces fat cells in the subcutaneous tissues, renders skin soft and flexible, increases circulation of the blood, stimulates activity of the skin glands, strengthens muscle fibres, refreshes and soothes nerves and relieves pain.

Massage —The Magic of Hands

The word massage was derived from the Arabic word *masah* which means the magic of hand. Massage is one of the easiest way of attaining and maintaining health, youth, vigour and beauty. Aches and pains, insomnia, tension and stress can be alleviated with a simple instrument—the hands. A touch of massage has great value in maintaining beauty and youth. Massage improves circulation, relaxes muscles, aids digestion by stimulating the lymphatic system, eliminates waste products, provides energy, refreshes and revitalises the body.

Early morning massage with hands provides miraculous effects in keeping body supple and healthy. Massage has been a popular medical treatment in Ayurveda and medicinal sciences. To have beneficial results, it is important that massage is given in a comfortable environment in a warm, peaceful place with dim lights, with the receiver of the massage lying on a firm surface with cushion under the knees, waist and neck to reduce the arch of the lower back and head. A soothing massage leaves one relaxed and asleep after finishing massage. As for the masseur, (the one giving the massage), follow these instructions: Keep your back straight throughout the massage, your feet wide apart and bend knees to give rhythm and depth to massage. Never stay in one position for long while massaging. Wear loose fitting, washable clothes and be barefoot. Remove all jewellery before giving massage which can cause scratches on the skin. Exercising the hands regularly before massage increase their sensitivity and flexibility. To keep the hands supple and fingers relaxed, rotate and stretch each finger and thumb in each direction one by one, then pull it gently with other hand. A firm, brisk massage is invigorating whereas slow, steady massage strokes can lead one to sleep.

Important Tips for Massage

- A rhythmic massage sends waves of relaxing throughout the body.
- Mould your hands to the contours of the body.
- Vary pressure from very light to very strong. The massage should be lighter over the bony areas and firmer over muscles.
- Do not apply heavy pressure when massaging.
- Avoid talking when doing massage.
- Cotton seed oil is most commonly used for massaging.
- Massage helps in dispelling headaches and migraines.
- Massage on the back should be the first area to start followed by massage of the feet which helps to relax the whole body. The whole body massage (including face and head) should take about 60 minutes.

Massage with Aromatic Oils

Massage with essential oils is very useful for the skin, and promotes vigour and vitality. For excessive oily skin use talcum powder for a dry massage. Use a light vegetable oil mixed with a few drops of essential oil for massaging. Pour about a teaspoon of oil into the palm of one hand, rub your hands together to warm it slightly and massage. Essential oils blended with massage oil add new dimension to massage. Essential oils have antibacterial, antiseptic or anti-inflammation properties and a right choice of oil leaves a calming and stimulating effect. Essential oils are extremely concentrated and must be diluted in a carrier oil while using them; otherwise they may cause allergies. The most common carrier oils are almond, soya, grape seed, avocado, peach and wheat germ oil. To dilute an essential oil, one to three drops are mixed to five teaspoons of carrier oil.

Oil		Properties and uses
Bergamot	:	Antiseptic, astringent. Used for acne and greasy skin.
Chamomile	:	Calming, soothing. Used for sensitive skins.
Clary Sage	:	Astringent, stimulating. Used as a fixative
Eucalyptus	:	Antiseptic, stimulating. Used for treating aching skin.
Frankincense	:	Calming, relaxing. Combats wrinkles and treats respiratory problems.
Geranium	:	Astringent, diuretic. Tones the skin.
Jasmine	:	Antidepressant, aphrodisiac. Good for beating postnatal depression and to speed up labour during child birth.
Lavender	:	Antiseptic, analgesic, calming. Treats aches, insomnia, depression and pains.
Marjoram	:	Analgesic, sedative, warming, comforting. Treats menstruation pain, aches and increases blood circulation.
Neroli	:	Sedative, calming. Suitable for dry skin, cures insomnia.
Petigrain	:	Sedative, calming, refreshing. Treats anxiety and insomnia.
Rose	:	Antiseptic, sedative. Very useful for skin disorders.

Rosemary	:	Stimulating. Treats rheumatic pain and aches.
Sandalwood	:	Antiseptic, sedative. Suitable for dry, dehydrated skins.
Tea Tree oil	:	Antiseptic, germicidal, fungicidal, soothing, healing. Treats infections, pimples, boils and burns.
Ylang Ylang	:	Antiseptic, sedative. Good for oily and problem skins.

Oils and Body Massage

Some women are born beautiful and others are not. Those who are born beautiful may look worn out with the passage of time and age. Oils play an important role, and their range is so vast that they cover the entire 'top to toe' beauty, body and hair treatments. There are three varieties of oils:

• Basic or original oils which are pure vegetable extracts.

• Processed or commercial oils prepared with analytical combinations of various necessary ingredients.

• Synthetic oils, whose use vary like their range.

To enhance beauty, almond, coconut, sesame, castor and olive are commonly used varieties of oils available in India. The following is some information regarding the cosmetic and pharmaceutical properties of these oils useful for skin and scalp.

Almond (Badam) Oil: There are two types: sweet and bitter. Bitter almond contains traces of hydrodynamic acid and is not recommended for beauty care. Sweet almond oil is used for face massage to improve complexion, prevent wrinkles around eyes, remove eye make-up, for dry and brittle hair, as body massage for dry skin and applied for healing of chapped lips.

Coconut (Nariyal) Oil: Oil is extracted from the dried kernel which contains 60 to 70 percent oil. The oil has benefits such as curing skin diseases, for thickness and growth of hair, curing leprosy wound, making hair healthy and lustrous.

Sesame (Til) Oil: Sesame seeds are of three types: White, red and black. The white seeds possess maximum oil. The oil extracted from black seeds has medicinal properties and contains 50 to 60 percent oil. It softens rough skin, good for growth of hair, is most beneficial oil base in formulations for massage in paralytic conditions, cleaning facial skin and massaging the body.

Olive (Jaitun) Oil: is a good conditioner, good for growth and thickening the hair.

Essential Oil Facial Massage

Massage of the face, neck and decollete area with essential oil is beneficial for several reasons:

- It stimulates the blood supply in the area, which increases the oxygen level and improves the tone of the skin.

- It increases the circulatory flow and the warmth created in the dermis by the massage movements allows greater absorption of the essential oils.

- It relaxes facial muscle tension, softening the facial expression under stress condition.

- It stimulates the lymphatic flow in the area, which can help speed up the elimination of cellular waste matter, toxins and other impurities including pollution.

- It helps dispel tiredness.

    The facial massage should be no longer than 20 minutes, and should be ideally between 10 to 15 minutes. The massage movement should be light but positive. The precise pressure used depends on the skin type—such as sensitive or allergenic. Each massage movement should be carried out 4 to 6 times depending on the skin type, age and the treatment being performed. Hands should always be relaxed and massage gently. Concentrate fully while doing massage, this assists the energetic flow from the hands.

Procedure for essential oil facial massage

This facial massage includes reflex points, holding movements, light effleurage and deeper tissue work, and is carried out on the neck and shoulders, as well as the face. Work on both sides of the face at the time. Follow the following steps:

- First, warm your hands by rubbing them together using light friction, and imagining warm energy flowing into them. This will help warm the massage oil.
- Pour a little of massage oil into the palm of one hand and rub both hands together.
- Gently press the oil on to the face, starting at the chin and working up the face in sections towards the forehead.
- Gently place your hands on the trapezius muscle, and in a continuous flowing movement using long strokes, move towards the occipital bone. Start with right hand, followed by the left hand. Repeat six times. Now wipe your hands.
- Pour a little of massage oil into your hands and use light effleurage movements, working upwards over the face.
- Starting at the middle of the sternum, use effleurage in a smooth movement towards the armpits, gradually moving upwards and outwards in sections until the

clavicle is reached. Use small circular travelling movements with the middle finger.

- Repeat these movements on the upper side of the clavicle, following the bone. Finish this movement by placing hands on both shoulders.
- Return to the face, and use effleurage movements.
- Starting at the centre of the chin, work upwards and outwards with your fingertips until the ear is reached. Use firm but gentle, small circular, stationary movements.
- Move up about half inch, and repeat the movements. Do this until the whole area under the lower lip is covered.
- Starting at the centre of the upper lip, work outwards with your index fingertip, finishing at the ear. Use gentle pressure, small circular, stationary movements, edging along one centimetre at a time. This is a repeating press-and-release movement. Moving upwards, repeat until underneath the cheekbone.
- Take the cheek muscle between your thumbs and index fingers, and gently squeeze.
- Rest for five seconds, resting both hands on the face. This movement aids energy flow.
- If incorporating reflex points into the massage, do this at this point.
- Smooth upwards along the sides of the face, starting at the chin and ending at the temples. Repeat three times; then smooth the forehead, towards the ears.
- Harmonise energy by holding the face in both hands for few seconds.
- Sweeping effleurage movements over the shoulders and neck. Repeat three times.

- At this point, any essential oil concentrate can be used. If treating conditions such as acne or sensitive skin, a compress or poultice may be needed.
- While your chosen extra product is left on the face, prepare a face mask.
- Apply the mask. Leave it on the face for approximately ten minutes.
- Remove the mask and apply a compatible moisturizer.
- Place both hands on the shoulders in the energy harmony position to a count of six.
- Relax for a few minutes, then make the receiver sit up and have a glass of water to drink.
- To complete the treatment, rub your hand briskly but gently up the vertebrae.

Essential Oil Massage

Apply essential oil diluted in vegetable carrier oil over the back, avoiding cellulite areas. Then apply the same massage oil, but at a 20 percent higher dilution, over the stubborn cellulite areas. Massage using movements that flow outwards and incorporate the pressing of the body's reflex points into the massage. Suitable essential oils to use in the massage oil are lemongrass, thyme linalol, rosemary, cypress, grapefruit, black pepper, juniper, fennel and eucalyptus.

Compress

To help increase circulation to stubborn areas, apply a ginger, black pepper and cardamom compress, wrapping the whole area of the body to be treated.

Skin brushing

It is to be carried out at least once a week.

Massage during Pregnancy

Essential oil massage can be very beneficial during pregnancy. Regular massage can even prepare the body for an easier delivery. Women having regular massage during pregnancy experience fewer tense muscles and become used to allowing the body to relax. Suitable essential oils during pregnancy include palmarosa, tangerine, geranium, camomile, roman, rose and jasmine. During labour, essential vapour can be diffused in the labour or delivery room.

There are few essential oils that cannot be used during pregnancy as hormonal and physiological changes take place during the period. These essential oils are annis, aniseed, basil, bay, birch, black pepper, cedarwood, cinnamon, cistus, clary sage, clove, cumin, fennel, no-leaf, hops, hyssop, juniper, lavendin, mace, marjoram, myrrh, niaouli, nutmeg, oregano, parsley seed, peppermint, pimento berry, rosemary, sage, spike lavender, spikenard, tarragon, thyme, valerian, wintergreen and yarrow. After careful choice of essential oils, use between 1/2 to 1 percent.

- To help support the breast, a small rolled towel or other support can be placed under the sternum. A soft pillow can be used for women with large breasts, and those with upper back and shoulder pain.
- Make sure to remove all clothes before massage, many women find this embarrassing but removal of clothes is conducive for better treatment.

Carry the Following Examination

Have the client sit on the couch with their back towards you, and

- Examine the vertebrae for any misalignments, redness or lumpiness.
- Note the posture. Are they leaning forward with the head hung down? Are the shoulders rounded?

- Smooth one hand over the whole of the back to feel how tense or stressed the muscles are. This will help in your choice of essential oils and help determine the body work technique that is required.

Carry our brief skin analysis to help choice of essential oils and body work techniques and see that:

- Pale skin indicates poor blood circulation or a medical condition such as anaemia or low blood pressure.
- Discoloured areas of body may indicate toxicity or previous bruising.
- Yellowish skin may indicate kidney problems or liver conditions.
- Bluish tinge may indicate poor blood circulation.
- Cold hands and feet may indicate poor blood circulation.
- Varicose veins may indicate colon problems, back problems, lack of exercise, stagnant energy and fluid flow.
- Spongy tissue may indicate water retention or poor nutrition.
- Tension in the muscles may be caused by injury, stress or holding the body in a fixed position.
- Knotted fibrous tissue may indicate scar tissue or congestion.
- Hard and congested areas on the body may indicate crystallisation.
- Thickened toe nails may indicate fungal, rheumatic condition.

Shiatsu Therapy

This therapy, also known as acupressure, is used to treat disorders by pressing various pressure points on the skin. There are nearly 600 shiatsu points in the human body and we shall discuss few very important ones. Pressure on such points produces energy that flows in the body and cures diseases. Shiatsu treatments are given on the floor. Make the receiver of the massage lie face down on a towel. Keep both hands moving rhythmically along the meridians from one point to the other pressing on each point for three to seven seconds. When breathing out, run down either side of spine. It takes about 45 to 60 minutes to treat the whole body, and it improves blood circulation and induces relaxation. The following steps are carried out while administering practice shiatsu:

• Press down either side of the spine.

• Use the heels of hand, then repeat with thumbs.

• Press down the buttocks and the back of the legs with light pressure over the knees.

• Squeeze down pressing in the points on the arms and hands, and the front of the legs.

• Press gently on all points in the abdomen working clockwise in circles.

• Work from the centre of the chest outwards, pressing in lines between the ribs.

Important Shiatsu Points on the Body

TABLE - I

Shiatsu points in the front portion of the body are illustrated in the figure below. The corresponding organs receiving the therapy and the beneficial effects are as follows:

1. Lungs and Chest. Relieves cough

2. Eases tension

3. Soothes tired arm and hand muscles. Dispels nervousness.

4. Alleviates body pain and restores energy.

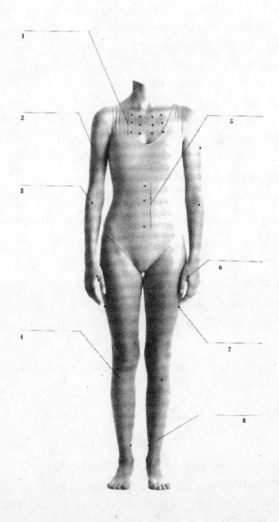

5. Alleviates menstrual problems and constipation.
6. Dispels pain and headaches (pregnant women should avoid).
7. Stimulates circulation and relaxes tired legs.
8. Eases menstrual pain and labour problems.

TABLE - II

Shiatsu Points in the back portion of body are illustrated in the figure below:

1. Dispels headache, backache and fatigue
2& 9 Dispels headache, cold, sinus problems and nosebleed.
3. Strengthens heart, lungs, digestion and reproductive organs.

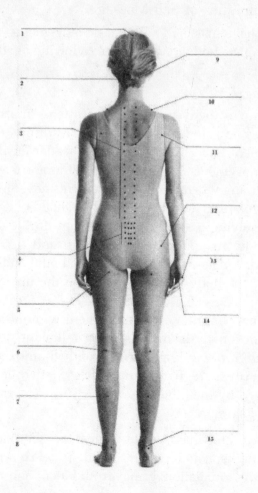

4, 8 & 15 Mensturation pain and backache.

5&7 Relieves back pain and tired legs.

6. Removes stomach pain and relaxes body.

10&11 Addresses headache and stiff shoulders.

12. Removes tension in the lower back.

13. Removes headache

14. Dispels nervousness and stimulates energy.

Basic Techniques of Self-Massage

Once you have mastered a few basic movements, you can give a complete body massage. The following are the basic movements used in massage.

- *Stroking:*

  It improves the circulation, relaxes tense muscles and soothes jangled nerves. This rhythmic flowing movement is a very common application in massage. Slow movements (applied by the palms and finger tips) are calming whereas brisk movements are stimulating. *Fan Stroking* is done by gliding both hands side by side and applying a steady, even pressure to the shape of the body. Avoid dragging the skin and keep hands relaxed. *Circle stroking* is used with both hands on one side of the body pressing firmly on the upwards and outwards stroke in wide circles. *Cat Stroking* is a soothing, soporific, slow movement without applying pressure on the skin, one hand following the other. *Thumb Stroking* is performed with thumbs applying slight pressure firmly upwards, with one thumb followed by the other.

- *Kneading:*

  It is a useful massage movement on shoulders, hips and thighs using plenty of oil. It relaxes muscles, improves circulation, brings fresh blood, and nutrients to the area and eliminates waste products. Basic kneading movements are *rhythmic* (pressing with the palm of one hand, grasping the flesh between the fingers of other hand), *wringing* (a deeper and more stimulating movement and administered as if you are wringing out a towel) and *light kneading* (done on less fleshy areas).

- *Pressure:*

The movement applying pressure releases tension in the muscles. This movement is especially useful when applied on spine and around the shoulders. Use little oil to enable hands slide smoothly.

- *Knuckling:*

The small circling strokes give a ripping effect when applied with the fists of curling hands. This massage movement is useful for massaging shoulders, chest, palms, hands and soles of the feet.

- *Percussion:*

Brisk, bouncy movements. Usually on fleshy, muscular areas of the body. Do not apply movement on bony areas, broken veins and bruises. The movement improves the circulation, has a calming effect and stimulates the nerves.

- *Cradling:*

It is a warming movement done with relaxed hands.

- *Criss Cross movements:*

Glide with both hands across the skin.

- *Cat Stroking:*

This smooth, slow, rhythmic movement calms the nerves leaving hypnotic, soporific effect. This movement is useful for massaging the neck, back, spinal area and bottom.

- *Feather Touch:*

  This light stroke rhythmic movement with both hands using finger tips leaves beneficial effect on the body.

- *Pummelling Stroke:*

  Pummel all over the skin with loose fists of flexible and loose hands which leaves stimulating and relaxing effect.

- *Final Touch Movement:*

  It is a finishing touch to massage with relaxed slightly cupped hands. Hold for some time and feel the heat seep into the body. Lift hands slowly.

Back Spine Massage

Back massage relaxes the spinal system. The spine is built of small bones called vertebrae. The spinal cord is a bunch of nerve-fibres running down through the spine. Start with stroking movement on the lower back, thumbs on either side of the spine and fingers pointing towards the head with relaxed hands. Now glide hands lightly downwards. Fan stroking, kneading, circle stroking and pressure stroking are various movements to bring blood to the nerves.

Neck and Shoulder Massage

Neck massage is essential as the nerves of this region have to support the weight of the head weighing between five to seven kilograms. The shoulder muscles usually remain tense. Neck massage includes the following movements.

- *Stroking :* Starting from the top of shoulders up towards the side of the neck gliding hands downward with smooth and even pressure. Kneading the neck muscle gently working from shoulders to the base of skull to ease tension. Circular Pressure movement is applied in circle upto the neck on either side of the spine with the fingers and thumb. This will relieve mental tension.

Buttocks Massage

Muscular tension generally exists at the lower back and buttocks. Buttocks muscles can be rid of tension with powerful massage movements as follows:-

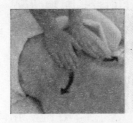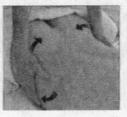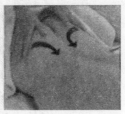

- *Circle Stroking :* with rhythmic strokes clockwise on right and anti-clockwise on left buttock.
- *Fan stroking :* fan stroking with relaxed hands smoothly in the upward direction far from the waist upward kneading fleshy buttocks.
- *Pressure movements :* Applying circular pressure with the thumbs of both hands at the bony base of the spine.

Foot Massage

Foot massage not only relaxes thousands of nerve endings in the sole but also refreshes and stimulates the whole body. The feet has as many as 28 separate bones and large number of muscles which help the foot to support the weight of the body and provide leverage when walking. The following strokes are applied during foot massage.

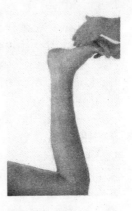

- *Stroking:* Start massage by stroking the feet from toes towards the ankles and back. Repeat 4-5 times.
- *Thumb Stroking:* Stroke up the foot with thumb from toe gliding to massage upto the ankles.

- *Toe Massage:* Rotate the hands wiggling the toes. The following three massage movements are to be given : Pressure is applied firmly on the sole holding the foot for 5 to 7 seconds. Work all over the ball of the foot. Stroking arch movements stimulate and soothe the foot by stroking the ball of the foot. Knuckling movement is applied keeping one hand on the top of the foot, stroking firmly all over the sole. Rotary pressure is applied by stroking the whole foot in circular upward pressure movement on sides all over the foot vigorously. Finally glide your hands slowly towards toes 3-4 times. In hacking movement hold the foot firmly with one hand and hack the sole with the side of other hand. To administer passive movements, support the ankle with one hand, loosen the muscle of foot and ankle with gentle passive movement with the other hand and slowly flex the foot up and down 4 to 5 times in each direction.

Leg Massage

Legs carry the weight of the body; hence they must be sturdy with strong muscles and bones. The knee joint is strengthened by the knee cap, a circular bone which helps the knee to carry the weight of the body. Deep, firm massage on the leg muscles helps to dispel fatigue, brings blood and nutrients to the leg muscles, relieves tightness or cramps and helps to prevent varicose veins. In case of varicose veins, massage gently, avoid heavy movements, such as kneading and pummelling. Gently stroke up the legs in the direction of lymph nodes (which exist at the back of knees and in the groin). This helps to reduce puffiness, swelling, aches and pain. Leg massage lying on the back is beneficial. Movements beneficial for the massage include:

- Stroking over ankles on sides of leg.

- Pressing toward the thighs.
- Kneading and squeezing ankles and calf muscles till the hands glide to and fro between knee and ankles.
- Stroking smoothly and firmly up the calf.
- Criss-cross movement on the calf muscles to release tension (avoid this movement in case of varicose veins).
- Stroking the thighs firmly between the hips and knee by criss crossing movement on thigh and squeezing in all directions.
- Thumb circle and rotary pressure stroking should be applied on thighs.
- Rolling and pinching the flesh over the outer thighs with thumb and fingers to release tension and improve skin texture.
- Passive movement over the knee and hips gently after massage has been finished, continue with knuckling movement (curling your hands into loose fists) for providing extra relaxing effect on thigh muscles.
- The movements for massaging back of the legs are similar to those used for massage of the front of the legs. For massaging back of the legs kneading and stroking-up movements are applied over the knee, thigh and calf.

Hand Massage

Hands are one of the most sensitive parts of the body which contain largest nerve endings linked to the brain to register sensation in the whole body. To ease stiff and tired muscles of the hand, a regular hand massage is a must. If neglected, skin of hands becomes aged and wrinkled easily due to lack of fat. Massaging hands with cream or oil stimulates the blood supply and keeps hands soft and supple. Hand massage can be given anywhere without inconvenience of getting undressed. Stroke the palm with the heel of other hand, thumb stroking towards the wrist and stretching the fingers are common movements for a hand massage. Fingers need massage. To work on each finger, stroke from the tip to the knuckle, followed by squeezing. Do apply circular pressure on each joint of the finger with the thumb. The following movements are suggested for hand massage:

- Stroke in the furrows between the tendons and wrist.
- Move fist all over the palm making rippling, circular movements with the knuckles of your fingers.
- Stretch the palm after you interlock your fingers in it applying circular pressure massage to ease tension from the hands.
- Give wrist massage holding the hand in the fingers. Stroke towards the arm.
- To give a final finishing touch to the hand massage, apply stroking movement on the whole hand for few seconds. Then release pressure by relaxing hand sliding slowly off the fingers.

Arm Massage

The bones of the arm and hands are more delicate than those of the legs and feet. Tension and tiredness in the arms lead to headache, neck pain and arching shoulders. A regular arm massage alleviates many body disorders. The techniques of arm massage are similar to those used in leg massage. For arm massage, start with a stroking movement across the wrist with slightly cupped hands to exert deep pressure on the muscle and light pressure over the bones. Glide your hands lightly downward on the sides of arms upto the wrist. Stroke up the forearm upto shoulders. Then glide downward. Fan stroking is conducted on the inside of the wrist. Clasp your hand around the wrist to drain out waste products from the veins.

The Forearm Massage

Kneading movement ensures that the arm is totally relaxed. Resting hand on the thighs knead the forearm gently working from wrist to elbow and back with both hands.

Elbow Massage

Stroke elbow smoothly with the tips of your fingers. Apply circular pressure. Finish massage by stroking movement to soothe the skin.

The Upper Arm Massage

Stroke the arm from elbow upwards to the shoulder. Pressing gently knead the upper arm with both hands together wringing and squeezing the flesh without hurting or pinching with a gentle pull. Make a large circle with the upper arm to rotate the shoulder joint which makes the arm fully relaxed.

Abdomen Massage

It calms the nerves and stimulates the digestive system. Abdomen massage relieves constipation, dissolves extra fat and improves skin texture. Usually, pregnant women are advised against abdomen massage but a very gentle abdomen massage is beneficial for the mother as well as child in womb. Movements such as stroking, circle stroking, rotary pressure, kneading, back lifting and feather stroking are recommended for abdomen massage.

Neck, Shoulders and Chest Massage

Poor posture and round shoulders make chest muscles tense. Bad sitting posture, long driving, horse riding, sports and respiratory diseases (asthma) all put strain on these muscles. Massage can help to stretch and relax the chest muscle, alleviate arching in the upper back, the neck and shoulders. Stretching and stroking movements are undertaken to massage neck, shoulder and chest. Start massaging with hands below the collar bones at the base of neck with smooth and firm pressure. Knuckling, deep pressure, kneading and alternate stroking are some of the massage movements to release tension. The muscles of neck are often taut and tense. The following movements stimulate blood flow and unknot tension.

- *Alternate Stroking:* With alternate hands stroke from shoulders to the skull base.

- *Side Stretch:* Cup one hand over shoulder and other at the base of the skull on the same side and stretch gently.

- *Pressure Stroking:* Exert firm, circular pressure on both sides of spine with middle fingers of each hand. Now press firmly over the skull base.

- *Passive Movement:* Avoiding jerking or pulling, smoothly cup hands at the base of skull and move to the neck with cupped hands. Gently move the forehead up and down as well as on sides until head moves freely.

- *Extra Movement:* Slide both hands as far under the back as possible. Pull the back. Be careful to avoid straining your back and arms.

Face Massage

For face massage, rhythmic strokes should be started with hands. Face massage improves your appearance, complexion, and prevents lines and wrinkles. Always use a fine quality oil on the face. Brisk and fast movements have an energising effect whereas slow and smooth movements are calming. Start at the base of neck to chin, move towards under the jaw to the ears, work back down under the chin. Continue stroking all over the face gliding from chin to the nostrils, the sides of the nose, below the eyes, under the cheek bones, upto the temples and back down the chin. Stroke again up to the bridge of the nose, then across the forehead to the temples and glide down to the chin. Cup your hands over the face and massage the forehead, press down, hold for few seconds, then release the pressure and remove hands. Repeat four to five times. Continue neck massage stroking from the shoulder to the neck and ears. Stimulate the jaw line by patting and slapping under the chin, under the jawline. Finally, soothe the massaged skin with gentle stroking.

Massage the cheeks, making circular, smooth, upward movements all around the mouth with loose fingertips. Stroke on the upper lip, under the cheek bones, around the ears, lower lip to the ears, cheeks and the jaws. Massage forehead and apply pressure with fingers. These soothing movements reduce tension and headaches. Upward circular movements energize whereas downward circular movements provide relaxation, soothe away tension and headaches.

To erase lines and wrinkles under and around the eye, start at the bridge of the nose, stroke lightly along the eyebrows with your fingertips, glide towards temples then back to under eyes and to the nose. Eye massage relaxes and dispels anxiety and tension. Squeeze the eyebrows between your thumbs and forefingers during the eye massage. As a finishing touch to the facial massage, cup your hands over the forehead. Hold, press down gently, then release the pressure slowly. Remove hands from the forehead. This will pull out tension from body.

Facial Reflex Points

Pressing reflex points as a part of facial increases energy flow and leads to revitalisation. The movements are carried out at the end of a facial:

- Press each of the points in sequence for a few seconds each. The movement is a gently press and lift, then release.
- Both sides of the face are treated at the same time.
- The first movement involves pressing in a continuous line.

The Movements

1. Start on the bridge of the nose, between the eyes, at the bottom of the forehead. Stroke in a continuous line straight up, to the centre of the hair-line, using both thumbs, one following the other. Repeat several times.

2. Start above the eyebrows, at the centre of the face. Press along the line of eyebrows. Again, at the centre, move up about 3/4 of a centimetre, and repeat the movement, working outwards. Carry on in this manner, until the whole forehead has been covered.

3. Smooth out both sides of the forehead, using all the fingers of both hands. Start at the centre and smooth outwards towards the temples.

4. Place both hands on the forehead, and hold for a count of six.

5. Starting under the inner eyebrows, press in a line working outwards.

6. Press adjacent to the outer corner of the eyes.

7. Start either side of the bulbous part of the nose, work outwards towards the ear. This first line should be under the cheekbone. Repeat, moving upwards until the whole of the upper cheek is covered.

8. Smooth over the upper cheekbone, then the lower cheekbone. Work from the centre, outwards. Both movements should end at the temples.

9. Starting above the side of the mouth, press in a line, outwards under the cheekbone. These points will involve lifting the flesh, and touching the cheekbone. Finish at the ear lobe.

10. Starting in the area between the nose and upper lip, use two fingers to press outwards in a continuous line. Repeat several times.

11. Starting under the lower lip, use two fingers to press outwards in a continuous line. Repeat several times.

12. Pinch gently along the jawline, working outwards.

13. Press along the entire hair-line, starting at the middle and working towards the ear. Repeat several times.

14. Using both hands, smooth upwards over both side of the face, then over the forehead, up both sides of the neck and into a classic shoulder and neck finish.

There are several extra reflex points on the face, which can be inserted at any time while performing a facial massage. This helps to improve the circulation and energy flow in the face, and also the tone of the skin. Hold each point for five seconds. These points are situated on the face/hands:

- At the centre of lower cheekbone, if the face looks tired or is sagging. This should be performed on both sides of the face.

- Either side of the nose, in line with the inner corners of the eyes, which helps reduce sinus problems and puffy eyes.

- At the outer corners of the eyes on both sides of the face, if the face looks tired or is sagging.

- In the middle of the eyebrows; this will encourage bodily energy flow and calmness.

- In the hollows just below the ears on both sides of the face, which helps droopy cheeks and jowls.

- On the border between the eye sockets and cheekbones in the middle on both sides of the face, which helps to tone cheek muscles and lift the face. This reduces the eye bags.

- At the centre of the palms of both hands, which generally energises the whole body.

Head Massage

A good brushing keeps the hair alive and provides it lustre. But a regular hair massage is an essential part of hair care. Scalp massage stimulates and increases blood circulation, removes hair dandruff flakes, relieves mental tension (if done on sections and nape of the neck), helps healthy growth of hair, if done near temples and the sides of the scalp). It not only stimulates the roots of the hair but also keeps facial muscles strong. Our hair is a chain of molecules held together that supply nourishment i.e., oxygen and food to the hair roots and carry away carbon dioxide and other metabolic waste material. When the waste products accumulate in the tissues, the blood circulation becomes poor and the growth of hair becomes slow and even ceases. For hair massage generally cotton, olive, coconut, mustard, almond oils are used. Head massage provides relaxation to every part of the body. The steps used for a scalp massage are as follows:

- Remove jewellery, brushing hair thoroughly, section the hair into half inch sections.

- Rub oil on each section of scalp and do scalp massage with the pressure of five finger tips (relaxing and smoothing). Manipulations for scalp massage include effleurage (stroking), patrissage (kneading), friction (rubbing), tapotment (percussion) and vibration (rapidly shaking or trembling).

Effleurage is introductory manipulation used on hair line applying pressure on various blood vessels which leave relaxing and soothing effect. The massage movement increases the blood circulation and strengthens the scalp tissues. Petrissage is an important scalp manipulation which involves light or heavy kneading, rolling, squeezing, pinching movements in circular motion to increase blood circulation in the scalp. Vibration is a rapid manipulation done with finger tips and palms which stimulates and relieves mental tension, disorders of scalp, cures baldness, makes the hair soft and supple, gives shine and nutrition to the hair. Tapotment movement consists of stroking the scalp and helps increase blood supply. This movement should not be done in case of high blood pressure and heart disease. Few head massage movements are described below.

- *Rotary pressure:* Massage in circles all over the scalp with pads of the fingers, this helps to release tension in the muscles.
- *Pulling the hair:* Stroke for sometime; then pull a bunch of hair. This movement relieves tightness in the scalp.
- *Massaging ears:* Squeeze the ears making circular pressures.
- *Stretching neck:* Massage behind the neck gently stretching the skull.
- *The finishing touch:* Place your hands on either side, fingers covering the ears. Gently press your hands, then release the pressure.

Self-Massage of Thighs and Legs

Leg massage can relieve aching caused by prolonged standing. Following steps are advised for a self-leg massage which helps tired muscles relax, stimulates the circulation of blood and the lymphatic system. Start stroking the whole leg from ankle to thigh beginning at the foot, up the calf, over the knee and up to the top of thigh, moulding hands to the shape of the legs and thigh. Knead thigh, rhythmically squeezing, then releasing the flesh. This helps to improve the shape and texture of the leg. Pummel the thigh with loosely clenched fists of hands which relieve stiffness in nerves. Stroke your knees softly with circular pressure massage. Finally, knead your calf muscle squeezing with both hands without exerting pressure on the bone.

Self Foot Massage

Foot problems lead to bad posture, backache and weariness. You can relieve tiredness, exhaustion and tension by regular feet and hands massage. Start massaging under the sole. Stroke smoothly from toes to your ankle and back to toes. Squeeze and stretch each toe. Press centre of the sole with thumbs giving circular motion around and on the ball of the foot. Do knuckling movements all over the sole in circles. Hack the sole with the ends of your hand. Stroke the ankles with fingertips and reverse all movements.

Self Hand Massage

Work the following movements : Stroke your hand towards the wrist gently. Squeeze each finger applying pressure over joints. Stroke between tendons on the back of hands. Apply static pressure all over the palm with thumb. Finish massage by stroking the palm with fingers.

Self Arms Massage

Thorough arm massage helps to dissolve tension in arms and shoulders, refreshes and soothes nerves. Stroke from wrist to shoulder. Glide back. Knead upper arms squeezing and releasing fleshy area. Apply circular pressures on forearm with thumb. Pat upper arm to stimulate circulation in muscles. Finish massage stroking your whole arm.

Abdomen and Hips Self massage

It provides comfort, and energy to the whole body. Lie down with your knees bent up stroke abdomen clockwise with both hands open. Knead all over abdomen with thumb and fingers. Then roll onto your stomach and knead hips and bottom. Cup your hands over your navel until you feel the heat, then lift slowly to release the pressure. Pummel your hips and bottom vigorously with loosely clenched fists.

Neck and Chin Self-Massage: The following movements stimulate the circulation, keep neck looking attractive and prevent development of double chin:

- Stroke from the collar bone to chin. Pinch along jaw line, starting from chin to the ears. Slap gently under the chin with hands to stimulate chin muscles.

- Stroke from the corners of your mouth towards ears. Press on the temples, clenching your teeth to stimulate the muscles and strengthen jaw.

Under-eye Massage : To dissolve lines and wrinkles under the eyes, following massage movements should be tried :

- Stroke gently with middle finger in circle around eyes from the bridge of nose out over eyebrows, pressing on the temples.

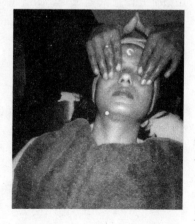

- Pinch along eyebrows from the centre to the temples with thumbs and index finger, pressing the bone under the eyebrows at the bridge of nose.

Massage for Expectant Mothers

Careful, smooth and gentle body massage movement benefit during the period of pregnancy. Massage helps alleviate many complications such as tension, backache, insomnia

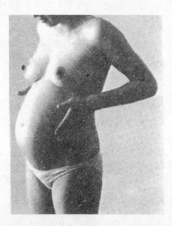
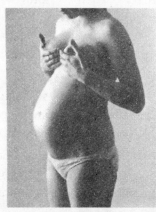

and fatty deposits on the body. Avoid deep pressure and percussion. A careful massage is definitely beneficial during pregnancy and before conception to increase the fertility of a woman. Use all stroking techniques described for abdomen, back, shoulder, leg and foot massage ensuring very gentle and light strokes. Massage done by a trained masseuse makes childbirth easier. Lower back and shoulders are the areas to concentrate for relieving tension while massaging. The various massage movements for a pregnant woman include gentle stroke on the abdomen with hands, one following the other clockwise. Stroke softly on the sides of the stomach based upwards with hands one following the other till hands reach the navel. Then glide hands gently towards abdomen. Cup your hands over the navel for few seconds until you feel the heat, then lift hands slowly.

Leg massage during pregnancy is especially beneficial, soothing, relaxing, relieving swelling and pain in legs. Varicose veins or cramps in the leg muscle are often faced by expectant women. Such women should always sleep with legs and feet slightly raised above the level of head. This correct sleeping posture relieves swollen legs by aiding manual lymph drainage. The lymphatic system drains off the waste products from the body. The lymphatic pumping system ensures healthy environment in body cells which fitter out waste products and bacteria from the blood and circulate purified blood in the body. Massage helps in pumping the lymph eliminating the waste from the body and strengthens the immune system curing many skin disorders like acne, eczema, dermatitis and inflammation of skin. Arm massage leaves soothing effect on the body when restrictions on abdomen massage are advised for expectant mothers. Backache and morning sickness are the common complaints during pregnancy and can be relieved to a great extent with back massage. Avoid deep pressure to the lower back. Back pain can be alleviated with plenty of smooth and flowing stroking movements on the mid back just above the waist at the base of spine and between shoulder blades. Press firmly applying circular pressure with your thumb on the hips and buttocks.

Massage after Child Birth

Massage to abdomen for 40 days after the delivery of baby, energizes the mother, cures body aches, sheds extra flesh and brings uterus to the original position prior to delivery. To give an abdomen massage to women after childbirth the following steps should be applied : Stroke the abdomen in all directions. Knead firmly on hips;

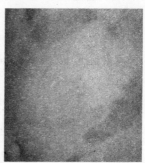

Wrinkles Spoty Abdomen

gently across the abdomen. Stroke clockwise in large circles on the abdomen. Apply gentle pressure clockwise on the abdomen. Stroke slowly up and on the lower abdomen starting from the pubic bone to the navel. Cup hands over the navel for few seconds until you feel heat under the hands, then lift hands slowly.

Massage Treatment for Weight Loss

Practise the following steps:

- Squeeze either side of the wrist above the wrist bone.
- Press on the hollow inside of the ankles just behind the bony prominence.
- Press in the middle of the groove between nose and upper lip.

To fight overweight, pay attention on the fleshiest areas of the body such as abdomen, thighs and buttocks using stimulating movements such as kneading and pummelling. Vigorous massage helps in slimming. Remember, massage alone (without regular exercise and control over the diet) cannot reduce weight or break down fat. Massage tones the skin, soothes the body, produces energy by stimulating the circulation. Weight watchers should concentrate on self massage of the following fleshiest areas :-

- *Abdomen:* Lie on your back and knead abdomen thoroughly.
- *Hips:* Roll on to one side; knead and pummel both hips.
- *Thighs:* Sit up and knead thighs from knee up to the hips vigorously.
- *Buttocks:* Pummel fast over thighs upto the buttocks.

Special Massage for Brides Before Marriage

Massaging with a massage cream has miraculous effect on the skin. A special recipe for brides to be used daily at the time of bath for ten days before marriage is to make a paste by mixing the following ingredients and rubbing it thoroughly to stimulate the skin leaving it soft and shiny. Mix 1 tbs dried ground lemon peel and almond, 4 tbs wheat germ flour, 1 tbs ground thyme, few drops of almond oil, jasmine oil and pinch of salt. Rub it on the body thoroughly for 30 minutes before taking bath daily.

CHAPTER–4

LINES AND WRINKLES

Ageing is the process When an individual grows old, the skin becomes dry as the sebaceous glands become less active. The skin loses its elasticity as the elastin fibres harden and wrinkles appear due to the cross linking and hardening of collagen fibres. The epidermis grows slowly and the skin appears thinner. Broken capillaries appear, especially on cheeks and around the nose. The facial contours become slack and muscle tone is reduced. Blood circulation slows down, which interferes with skin nutrition, and the skin may appear sallow. Metabolism slows down. Collagen production breaks down. Hormone production is reduced. Patches of irregular pigmentation appear on the surface of the skin. Dark circles and puffiness may occur under the eyes.

Lines and Wrinkles

Fine lines are shallow grooves in the epidermis which can be made to look less obvious by the use of cosmetic products that improve hydration and suppleness. Wrinkles are of two types : permanent and non-permanent. Permanent wrinkles are present as a deep wrinkle on sun-exposed skin, such as the face and neck and do not disappear on stretching. The other type is a fine, shallow wrinkle that develops on sun-protected skin, such as abdomen and bottom, where the skin becomes thin and wrinkles easily as subcutaneous fat tissues decrease with age; these wrinkles disappear easily on stretching. Cosmetic products cannot reverse wrinkle development as wrinkles are the effect of changes in the dermis.

As we grow older, fine lines and wrinkles begin to develop. The skin loses its firmness and elasticity. Expression lines on the face, and the patches of discolouration on areas of dilated blood vessels appear. The reasons for these changes are due to sluggish blood circulation and slow metabolism. Chemical changes take place in the tissues, sebaceous glands diminish in size and number (particularly in women), collagen production breaks down and hormone production is altered or reduced.

Smoking and Your Skin

It is wise to avoid smoking; it damages the appearance of the skin. Cigarette smoke and tar deprive the skin of the nutrients and oxygen it needs for good health, leaving it looking dull and lifeless. They lead to the formation of harmful free radicals and weaken the collagen and elastin fibres with the result that the skin becomes permanently wrinkled.

The Effect of Hormones

There is a relationship between beauty and hormones. The hormones are produced in human body by various organs. Lack of or excess of hormones or their imbalance can prove disastrous. Hormones are of various types, but the ones associated with ageing are androgens, estrogens, thyroids, steroids, insulin and sex hormones. *Androgens* are basically male hormones which are produced in the adrenal glands in women. Excessive secretion of androgens activate the production of sebum of the sebaceous glands causing acne or hair loss. The excessive secretion of androgens is usually caused by stress and mental tension. The imbalance of hormones must be diagnosed by a qualified doctor and may be balanced by taking estrogen pills. *Estrogens* are normally female hormones produced by the ovaries. These reduce the secretion of sebum and cure acne and pimples. Estrogen pills generally lead to gain in weight. Replacement of these hormones are essential for some women after the age of 40 when the production of these hormones decline. Therapy benefits the skin by retarding wrinkles and making it clear and shiny. Avoid taking estrogen pills, if you suffer from high blood pressure. In all cases, the therapy has to be prescribed by a medical doctor. Estrogen therapy sometimes harms the skin causing pigmentation or skin lesions. The shortage of *Thyroid hormones* secreted by thyroid glands makes the skin dry and wrinkled. Excessive production of steroids (by adrenal glands) causes skin infections, pigmentation and acne. The deficiency of *insulin hormones* harms the complexion and causes skin fungus such as bacterial infection and itching. *Sex hormones* are of two types—male sex hormones and female sex hormones. Male sex hormones encourage growth of hair on the skin and body, whereas female sex hormones encourage growth of hair on the scalp.

What Causes Wrinkles ?

As a person ages, skin cells divide more slowly, and the inner skin, or dermis, starts to thin. Skin loses its elasticity; when pressed, it no longer springs back to its initial position but instead sags and becomes dry and scaly. The ability of the skin to repair itself declines, so wounds are slower to heal. Frown lines (between the eyebrows) and crow's feet (lines that radiate from the eyes) appear; permanent small muscle contractions contribute to the formation of jowls and drooping eyelids. Wrinkles appear on the forehead.

Sun Damage (Photoageing)

The skin ages prematurely as a result of prolonged exposure to ultraviolet (UV) radiation from the sun. The role of the sun cannot be overestimated as 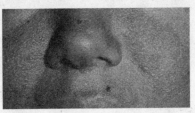 the most important cause of over ageing; skin exposure to ultraviolet (referred to as UVA or UVB) radiation from sunlight accounts for about 90% of the premature skin ageing and most of these effects occur by the age of 20. UVB is the primary agent in sun burning. UVA penetrates more deeply and efficiently. Both UVA and UVB rays cause damage leading to lower immunity against infection, ageing skin disorders, and cancer. Even small amounts of UV radiation damage major structural protein in the skin and cause accumulation of abnormal elastin (the protein that causes tissue to stretch). In this process, large amount of enzymes called metalloproteinases are produced. The normal function of these enzymes is to cure sun-injured tissue by synthesizing and reforming collagen. One study indicated that when people with fair skin colour are exposed to sunlight for just five to 15 minutes, metalloproteinases remain elevated for about a week. Other environmental factors, including cigarette smoke and pollution, may hasten chronological ageing process and skin cancer. Rapid weight loss can also cause wrinkles by reducing the volume of fleshy cushion. This not only makes a person look gaunt, but can cause the skin to sag.

How Can Wrinkles be Prevented?

Avoiding Intense Overexposure to Sunlight

The best way to prevent skin damage is to avoid episodes of excessive exposure of sun during the hours of 10 am to

4 pm. Ultraviolet intensity depends on the angle of the sun, not heat.

Sunscreens provide protection against skin cancers caused by the skin being exposed to harsh ultra violet rays from the sun. This hastens the process of ageing, causes wrinkles, skin burns and may finally cause skin cancer. Studies show that the sun emits two different ultra violet rays : UVA and UVB. The UVB causes sunburns, while UVA causes skin cancer. The beauty world was rocked in 1997 when UVA rays were detected in sunrays and found to cause different types of skin cancer. Compounds like Avonbenzone, Titanium Dioxide, Zinc oxide were found to protect and act as ideal ingredients for prevention of the disease. Indian skin types do not generally get sunburnt, but tan profusely. The fair skinned people generally use tanning lotions while the remaining are into fairness creams.

Daily Preventive Skin Care

As part of a regular routine, it is advisable to wash the face with a mild soap that contains moisturisers. Alkaline soaps should be avoided. The skin should be patted dry and immediately lubricated with a water based moisturiser. Many creams and lotions are available for wrinkle-protection, although very few have been proven to be effective. Soap that contains salicylic acid can help remove old skin. It is very important to rub gently. Rubbing perpendicular to the wrinkle, mechanically removes the outer layer of dead skin cells and is particularly effective. Exfoliation using scrubs, however causes certain conditions, such as acne, sensitive skin, or broken blood vessels.

Skin Rehydration Service to Combat Ageing

This service includes *skin cleansing,* a 75-minute skin treatment comprising a complete revitalization and cleansing with cream, steaming with plant essences, deep cleaning to remove impurities and a rejuvenation massage up to the neck. *Skin rehydration* is a 60-minute treatment to recondition tired skin through rehydration with vitamin creams, lotions and moisturizers; it refreshes, and restores the softness and elasticity of youth. *Skin nourishment* is a 60-minute treatment with face masks and specialised massage with creams and lotions to lubricate and revitalise the skin.

What to do in Case of Sunburn?

Take aspirin or paracetamol to reduce inflammation and control pain (with the consultation of doctor). Cool, wet compresses or cool socks for 15 to 20 minutes four to five times daily will control pain. Do not apply butter or heavy ointments on the burned skin as these cause skin irritation. Increased fluid loss can occur through badly sunburned skin. Fluid replenishment with an isotonic drink is recommended. Avoid more sun exposure until the skin completely heals. Sun-damaged skin is more susceptible to subsequent burns.

Why does Skin Age ?

Ageing of skin occurs as collagen and elastin, the two major components in the underlying support structure of the skin, degenerate. The major factor in this degeneration is ultra violets (UV) light from sun. Skin is also damaged by nasty little single molecules called free radicals, (generated during assimilation of junk food) which cause cellular havoc and the skin begins to line, sag and wrinkle. Sun exposure must be avoided where possible since much of the harm is done before the age of 18. From the age of 50, the number of elastin fibres declines tremendously, accelerating the dropping, bagging and sagging. At the same time, the skin becomes drier because oil production diminished, as does the skin's ability to hold water and the rate of cell renewal also reduces.

The Signs of Ageing

The average adult has some 300 million skin cells, covering upto 2 sqm of skin, weighing 3.2 kg. Facial skin is about 0.12 mm thick, body skin about 0.6 mm; and the thickest areas on palms and soles about 1.2 mm or more upto 4.7 mm. The thinnest skin is on the lips and eyes. Each square half inch of skin contains, on average, at least ten hairs, 100 sweat glands, tiny blood vessels and 15 sebaceous glands.

The loss of skin elasticity, increased wrinkles, sagging breasts and lack of skin firmness are all inevitable signs of ageing. Around and after the age of 40, skin cells begin to take longer to regenerate due to the change in hormones and decreasing levels of vitamin E. The following developments appear with each stage of life: The brain starts maturing rapidly by the age of three. The sex hormones start producing in the female body by the age of seven. The growth accelerates upto the age of puberty and starts to slow down until long bones stop growing, by the age of 20. A female becomes hyper fertile in early twenties and decline in her fertility starts when she reaches the age of 30. The height of a female starts to diminish between the age 30-40. The hair pigment cells in the scalp reduce their activities between the age of 40 to 50, leading to grey hair and hair loss. Lot of care is needed between 50 to 60 when the body begins to put on weight during the period of menopause. Between 60 to 70 the red blood cells start reducing in their body and their quality also begins to deteriorate. In the age of 70 to 80, spine starts to curves as the spinal disc shrinks and bones in the body become thin and weak. Between the age 80 to 90, the body loses seventy percent of the muscle mass as compared to youth (age of 30).

An Attractive Package to Look Young After 40

Laugh lines and grey hairs give obvious clues to a woman's age. Here are five steps to beat ageing :

- Wrinkled and sagging breasts are tell-tale signs of ageing; as we grow older, breasts start to lose their firmness and often get wrinkled, concave and develop stretch marks. The main factors affecting their shape are rapid weight loss or gain, pregnancy, breast feeding etc. Breasts are made up of fat, so any weight change affects their shape as the skin here is very soft. Exercising without a proper bra also causes stretch marks. Pregnancy causes breasts to sag. Even a woman with small breasts will find that her breasts grow extremely rapidly in pregnancy. Breast feeding is responsible for the concave look many women have in their upper breasts, it can leave them looking wrinkled and deflated. Correctly fitted bras and exercises to stimulate breasts can help build up the supporting area around the breasts. Swimming is a good exercise for breasts. Only surgery can make breasts look younger.

- The signs of ageing skin include loss of elasticity, increased wrinkles and lack of skin firmness. From around the age of 40, our skin cells take longer to regenerate due to hormonal changes and decreasing level of vitamin E. When we are younger, skin cells replenish themselves within 21 days but this rate becomes slower as we grow older. Deep penetrating aroma therapy oils stimulate the skin and promote its regeneration.

- Exfoliation encourages circulation and stimulates the skin and sloughs away any dead cells. Body brushing, too, stimulates lymph flow, helps detoxify the body and acts as an effective stimulant. Vigorous rubbing or pinching the skin promotes fine lines and encourages wrinkles. Moisturiser should be dabbed lightly and rubbed in gently. Cold shower can tone the skin and stimulate the nervous system.

- Hormone replacement therapy (HRT) can aid the skin's elasticity as estrogen helps to promote the production of protein collagen, which exists as thick fibres in the skin. However, HRT should be taken only under the prescription of a qualified doctor.

- In case of signs of ageing skin, women should avoid sunbathing. Women with darker skin tend to look younger for longer because they have a natural sun block. Excessive exercise after the age of 40 is harmful; as we get older, the skin cannot easily spring back into place, so do gentle stretching and light yoga postures only. Stretch marks on the body pose serious signs of ageing. Stretch marks are caused by scar tissue just below the skin's surface as a result of stress and strain on the skin. They are associated with pregnancy but can also occur with weight gain or at puberty, and once established, are almost impossible to eradicate. An effective way to fade stretch marks is to use vitamin E, which can regenerate damaged skin tissues. Wheat germ oil or vitamin E capsules should be cut open and used immediately causing scars to fade altogether. Pregnant women should apply wheatgerm oil every day to stomach, abdomen and breasts.

- Faulty posture causes signs of ageing. Rounded or hunched shoulders make you look older. It's vital to keep the spine supple. Standing with your weight on one leg, hunching over your working table, and stooping create havoc on your appearance as well as health. To overcome this problem and to keep your spine fluid, walk a couple of kilometers a day or swim regularly. Take up yoga or a keep-fit class. Avoid wearing high heels or shoes with excessively pointed toes. Sagging buttocks, too, are a sign of ageing. Slack, loose bottoms are the fate of many of us as we get older. The reasons for the sagging of bottoms are lack of muscle tone, lack of support and elasticity in the skin. A regular massage with anti-cellulite oils can help break down the fatty deposits underneath the skin. Do exercises specifically for the buttocks that involve clenching and unclenching the buttocks. You can have a face of 25-year-old, but wrinkles on vour hands will give away your real age. Hands do not have natural oils and due to improper moisturising, the skin begins to lose its elasticity. Mottled skin on the thighs indicates faulty circulation and can be improved with the help of a friction mitt used in a circular motion. A spotted back is often a problem for women. The back is usually the most neglected part of the body. The best remedy for this is to keep the skin scrupulously clean by washing with medicated liquid soap.

Aromatherapy for Internal and External beautification: Aromatherapy is fast gaining popularity as an 'alternative' or 'holistic' medicine, for the balance of body, mind and spirit. Derived from the ancient practice of using natural plant essence to soothe nerves and promote health, this therapy was initially primarily used to adorn bodies. A single drop of essential oil is equivalent to an ounce of a living plant, making the essence highly potent. This therapy works on the mind, through the pores of the skin. The plant extracts enter the body through inhalation or massage. Self-practice of aroma therapy without full know-how is not advisable as concentrated oils are very strong and can have diverse effects. Each aroma used must be acceptable to body for positive effect. Essential oils reduce or intensify mental activity. They are antiseptic, antibacterial, anti-viral, antitoxic and anti-inflammatory. The most common oils are grapeseed oil (all purpose carrier oil, as a base for massage), avocado oil, sweet almond oil, calendula oil—all for treating scars and blemishes and softening skin. Preparations made from essential oils and base liquids include cleansers (with strong antiseptic quality that helps remove trapped dirt, cleanse the skin and soothe inflamed areas, moisturisers (that reduce fine lines and help weatherproofing) and face oils which have good effect on the blemishes on combination skin, and help loosen dirt trapped in pores and rejuvenate dry and wrinkled skin by inducing relaxation.

Aroma Massage on Reflex Points

Massage the reflex points with small, 'stationary,' circular movements. Pressure should be applied for three seconds at each point on the important pressure points on the body as shown in the illustration below which slim, tone, energise and relax the body:

1. On the sole of the foot.
2. Behind the ankle bone.

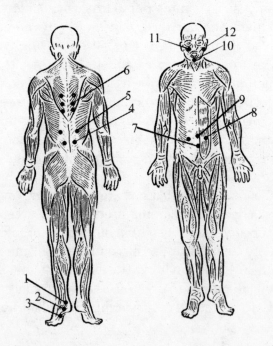

3. Ball of the foot.

4. On the back at waistline.

5. On the back, above waistline.

6. On the back on either side of vertebrae.

7. On the back, three inches below the navel.

8. One inch either side of the navel.

9. On four inches above the navel.

10. At the lower cheekbone on both sides.

11. On either side of nose.

12. The hollows below the ears.

CHAPTER–5

MAKE-UP TECHNIQUES

The face is the most attractive part of one's personality. Skilful make-up enhances its appeal and makes one look grooming and make-up, they become the centre of attraction. The basis of the art of skilful make-up is honesty. The woman who looks good despite facial faults is the woman who knows what those faults are. A careful assessment of facial shape and profile is the first essential step in using make-up successfully. The ideal make-up for you is the one that makes the best of your face. Know your face, sit in front of a mirror, remove make-up, now take a hand mirror and hold it in such a way that you can see the reflection of your face in the first mirror reflected in the second mirror. Skilfully done make-up enhances

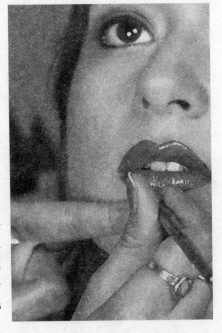

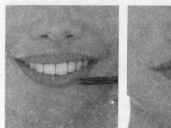 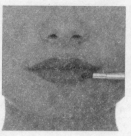 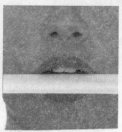

your appeal and gives you an added dignity in society and helps you gain self-confidence. It is therefore necessary to know the secrets of beauty aids, art of using them and thorough knowledge of various beauty products available in the market. It is helpful to apply a good foundation or lotion on hands, neck and face before make-up, so that the skin appears even. Powder gives a kind of glow to the cheeks, so does the cream. Rouge heightens the natural pink tinge of the cheeks. Eyes lend charm to the face. The beauty of eyes can be increased by eye make-up products, such as eye-shadow, eye liner and mascara.

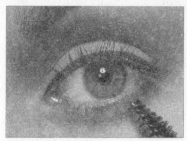 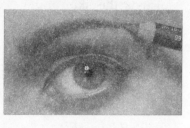

Wrong choice of make up may affect the skin, you may look unattractive or more aged than your actual age. In order to keep your facial skin young and glowing you can

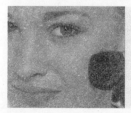 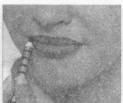 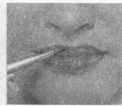

use cold cream, cleansing cream, astringent lotion, calamine lotion, foundation cream and face powder.

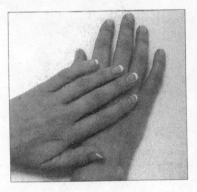 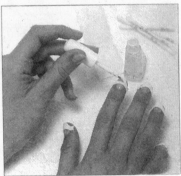

Cold cream

It is used to minimise the effect of cold climate and dry breezes. Cleans the skin of dust and dirt.

Vanishing cream

Moistens the skin and is beneficial for oily and normal skin. Vanishing cream provides a glow to the face, if used before make-up.

Nourishing cream

Softens the skin and keeps it glowing.

Cleansing Cream

It is used to clean the facial skin. It removes stale make-up, dust and sweat, resulting in wrinkles and dullness.

Astringent Lotion

It is used to open clogged pores of the skin.

Calamine Lotion

It is used to make skin even.

Foundation Cream

It makes the skin smooth and make-up appealing.

Face Powder

Makes the face look glowing and bright.

Types of Skin

Ivory Skin

Clear blemish-free creamy skin.

Olive Skin

Tans well in summer but looks sallow in winter.

Tawny Skin

Honey-coloured warm skin, tans easily to a rich colour.

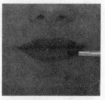

Florid Skin

Sensitive, fair skin, erupts with blemishes and freckles easily.

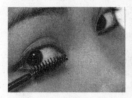 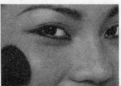 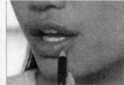

Art of Make-up

Applying foundation is a most important part of make-up. Foundation is an effective beauty aid to hide any spots on the face. And give an even look. It also makes the skin look attractive. Always clean your face with deep cleansing milk before applying the foundation. Shake the foundation

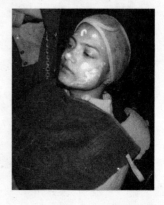

cream and apply as a dot over forehead, cheeks, nose, chin and neck, and massage with an upward motion to give an even look. Foundation is not only the base make but also a protective agent to hide pimples, shadows and spots on the face.

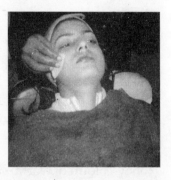

Apply powder to settle a foundation and give a smooth surface. It is your choice whether to use compact or powder. Choose the shade of powder according to your complexion so that it may settle with the skin colour. Apply powder with a clean puff. Dust off extra powder with brush.

Rouge is applied with brush. Use slightly, so that it should only give pinkish natural glow to cheeks. Cream rouge is applied on dry skin. Rouge is capable to change the shape of the face.

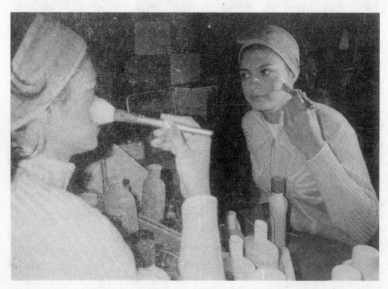

Making beautiful eyes

Applying foundation, eye shadow, mascara, eye brow pencil and eyeliner are various steps for making eyes beautiful. Apply lid shadow in light stroke, then crease shadow and

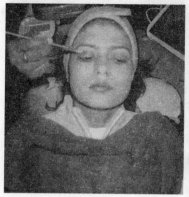
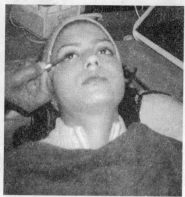

finally the shadow on the brow bone. Eye shadow is used on eyelids between eyebrow and eyelashes applied with fingers. Now apply mascara in upward strokes on top lash and downward stroke on the bottom one. Apply a coat and allow to dry, then apply second coat. Apply eye brow

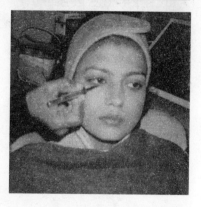

pencil lightly to give natural curve to the lashes. If the hair is brown, apply dark shade pencil. Now apply eyeliner, starting from inner corner of the eyes and extend to the outer corner. Eyes can be made to appear larger or smaller through eye shadow.

Lip colour

Dab a little cold cream to soften the lips if they are too dry. Draw a neat line following the natural lip line with thin lip

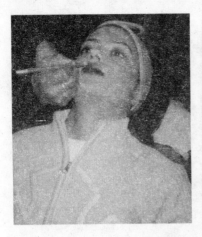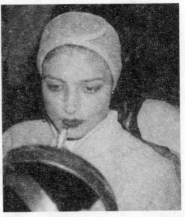

brush dipped in lipstick. Fill in lipstick with a thicker brush. Press on tissue paper to remove excess. Apply a thin coat of lipstick or lip glosser.

Do not forget to apply make-up on the neck, always treat it as face.

CHAPTER–6

DRUGLESS THERAPIES TO FIGHT AGEING

Hydrotherapy (Therapeutic Baths)

An important factor in the cure of diseases by natural methods is to stimulate the vitality of the body and fight ageing and obesity – by using water in various ways and at varying temperature in the form of packs or baths as described below. The process of application of water for treatment is known as hydrotherapy.

Cold Hip Bath

For chronic as well as general health problems and to reduce the fatness a cold hip bath is advised. While taking the bath patient should be given a wet cloth and should be directed to rub the abdomen from the navel downwards. The time period for the bath should be from 15 to 30 minutes with the water temperature between 10°C-20°C.

Hot Hip Bath

Immediately after the cold hip bath, hot hip bath is suggested to make blood circulation of the body fast. This bath also cures skin ailments. Always drink a glass of water before taking bath to maintain the moisture level of the body. The duration of bath should be 10-15 minutes at water temperature should be between 40°C-50°C.

Neutral Hip Bath

This bath is beneficial to give relief to inflammatory conditions of the different sensitive parts of body. A patient can have bath between 15 minutes to an hour at water temperature between 30°C-35°C.

Alternate Hip Bath

It is a hot and cold water bath simultaneously. The time period for the bath should be between 15-20 minutes. The temperature of hot water should be between 40°C-45°C and cold water 10°C-20°C. The alternate hot and cold water bath activates the blood vessels of the skin and treat the chronic inflammatory problems.

Cold and Hot Immersion Bath

As suggested by name before the bath, the patient should take a glass of water to retain body moisture. As after the bath skin of the body becomes dry, massage oil on the patient's body. Don't forget to wet head and neck before bath.

Epsom Salt Bath

This bath is useful before sleeping at night. Take a tub filled with hot water with temperature of 40°C and mix to it 1 kg of epsom salt. Lie in the tub putting your thighs and legs immersed in water for 20 minutes.

Hot and Cold Foot Bath

For this bath, feet are immersed in hot water at 40°C-50°C, followed by cold water with the temperature of 10°C-12°C.

Hot Foot Immersion

Immersion bath is administered in a bath tub fitted with hot and cold water connections. A hot foot bath stimulates the involuntary muscles of body. In this bath legs are immersed in a tub or bucket filled with hot water at temperature of 40°C-50°C. The duration of the bath is generally 10 to 20 minutes. Take cold shower immediately after the bath.

Mud Packs and Therapy

Mud therapy cures all skin problems. The clay is dug from deep earth for its purity as it contains healing properties. The part of clay mixed with warm water is applied on the body. It improves the complexion and helps to detoxify the matter. It also helps to maintain the moisture of the body and is an anti-wrinkle beauty treatment.

Spinal Bath

It is an important form of hydrotherapy treatment given in a special designed tub which provides a soothing effect to the spinal column and influences the central nervous system. The bath can be administered at cold, neutral and hot temperatures. The water level in the tub should be two inches above hips and the patient should lie in it for 3 to 10 minutes. The cold spinal bath relieves irritation, fatigue, hypertension, excitement and nervous disorders (hysteria, fits, mental disorders, loss of memory and tension). Neutral spinal bath for 20 to 30 minutes is a soothing and sedative treatment and relieves irritation. Hot spinal bath helps to stimulate depressed nerves, relieves vertebral pain in spondylitis and muscular backache.

Steam Bath

Steam Bath also known as sauna bath is a time tested water treatment which induces perspiration. Many questions arise.

Does sauna bath help to slim down? Is it good or bad for the skin? How long should one stay in the steam ? What dress to wear when having sauna bath ? In what position should one take this bath? Sauna can do wonders in reducing weight and clearing cellulitis. Sauna is a place to relax, to lie prone, speechless, to exercise 15 minutes in sauna is equivalent to running two kilometres. The dress worn at the time of sauna is generally bare body, in briefs and bras or swim suit. Bare body reaps more benefits than a covered one. Wrap hair in a towel or turban. Do not wear watch and jewellery when taking steam bath – the steam and heat shall damage them badly. A cold shower taken immediately after the bath is ideal. Sauna bath eliminates toxins through the skin, relieving acne, brightening dull lifeless complexion.

The Hot Air Bath

It consists of exposure of the entire body (except head) to a superheated atmosphere. The air in a specialised cabinet is heated to the desired temperature of 48°C to 90°C, sufficient to produce profuse perspiration; drink a glass of water just before taking this bath. The cold application following the hot bath increases the tone of blood vessels, energises the nervous system and changes the condition of passive congestion of the skin. Do not employ high temperatures to those suffering from cardiac trouble. The hot air bath should be avoided in case of eruptive skin disorders, extreme cardiac weakness, in febrile conditions like diabetes, goitre, arteriosclerosis and advanced cases of nephritis.

The Turkish Bath

It is similar to the hot air bath in which the whole body is heated accompanied by friction, kneading of the muscles and shampooing in a room having chambers for dressing, a warm chamber or tepidarium (temperature 43°C to 54°C), calidarium or hot room (temperature 65.5°C to 76.5°C) and a shampoo room, and a chamber having douche apparatus, provision for a plunge bath and cooling arrangements. During the initial 10 to 12 minutes, the patient is frequently rubbed to induce perspiration. May apply a hot foot bath or a hot fomentation to the spine. When the patient begins to perspire, he/she should enter the hot room, then to the shampoo room. Rubbings and strokings are continued with firm pressure movement and rapid to and fro movements applied on arms, chest and abdomen etc. Avoid this bath in cases of organic disease of heart, kidneys and diabetes.

Graduated Bath

It is used for the treatment of fevers. The initial temperature of the bath should be one or two degrees below the temperature of the body of the patient. The temperature of water is cooled after every five minutes until the temperature of bath drops by 75% to 80%. Avoid cold graduated bath in case of diseased/very weak heart.

Cold Friction

It involves the application of a series of wet rubbings to the surface of the body with the help of friction mitt and cold water (preferably ice cold). The patient is undressed, made to lie on the bed wrapped in a turkish towel. A sheet wet in cold water is rubbed on the patient's body on the trunk back of the legs, the back, the hips and the feet rapidly.

Juice Therapy (Juice Fasting)

It is the most effective way to restore health, rejuvenate the body and regain lasting youth. Raw juice therapy is a method of treatment of disease through an exclusive diet of fruit and vegetable juices. Drinking alkali forming fruit and vegetable juice during fasting increases the healing effect of fasting by eliminating uric acid and other inorganic acids. A glass of water mixed with lemon juice and 20 to 30 grains of honey may be taken first in the morning, which helps to rejuvenate the skin. A patient should take adequate rest during the raw juice therapy. Fruit and vegetable juices beneficial in treating skin aliment are mentioned below :

For acne/pimples, have juice of grapes, pear, plum, tomato, cucumber and spinach. For skin allergies and anaemia, have apricot, grapes and carrot juice. Apple, beet and apricot juices cure constipation. Papaya, lemon, pineapple juices help in case of diarrhoea. In case of eczema and psoriasis skin disease, take carrot, spinach, cucumber and beet juices. Heart disease and hypertension are cured with the juice of grapes, lemon, cucumber, carrot and spinach. Women suffering from menstruation problem are advised to take grapes, orange, lemon, cherry, lettuce and spinach juice. Obesity is cured with lemon, grapefruit, orange, carrot and cabbage juice. Piles are treated with lemon, orange, papaya, trump, pineapple juices. In case of suffering from varicone veins have grape, orange, tomato, carrot and watercress juices.

Chromotherapy and Ageing

The sun looks white, but has seven colours, violet, indigo, blue, green, yellow, orange and red. Chromotherapy is very effective for chronic and dreaded diseases. Exposing a diseased body part to sunrays passing through coloured glass, 90 minutes after sunrise and 60 minutes before sun set has a curative effect. Keep the glass of desired colour in the sunlight in such a way that the rays pass through it and fall on the affected parts. While receiving sunlight therapy, care should be taken that the patient is not exposed to strong direct wind. If sunlight is not possible, take a 60 to 100 watts coloured bulb. In case such coloured bulb is not available, take a plain bulb and wrap coloured gelatine paper around it. Keep affected part about 20 inches away and have the light shine on it for 5 to 10 minutes twice a day.

To practise chromotherapy-water therapy take a glass bottle of the desired colour or wrap gelatine paper of the desire colour on white glass bottle. Fill it 3/4th with water and keep it in sunlight for at least three hours between 10 a.m. and 3 p.m. Take care, the coloured water is not exposed to any other type of colours. The colour-medicated water can be given to the patient at an interval of 15 minutes to two hours depending upon the intensity of the disease The effect of different colours on various skin disorders and ageing is listed below:

Violet cures diseases of bones and baldness. Indigo cures eye- nose-throat problems, facial paralysis, diseases of lungs, asthma, indigestion and problems of nervous system. *Blue* cures nervous disorders, measles, small pox, insomnia, mental depression, burns, semen discharge, premature ejaculation. *Green* cures heart troubles, liver disorders, high blood pressure, venereal disease and inflammation in eyes. *Yellow* cures disorders of digestion, spleen, liver problems, diabetes and leprosy. *Orange* cures asthma, bronchitis, gout, kidney swelling and mental nervousness, epilepsy. *Red* cures anaemia, sluggishness, paralysis, white spots, arthritis.

Enema Therapy

It is known as rectal irrigation; an enema involves the injection of fluid into the rectum. In nature-cure treatment, only lukewarm water with or without lime juice is used for cleaning the bowels. A hot water enema is beneficial in relieving irritation due to inflammation of the rectum and painful haemorrhoids. An enema with warm water, 1 to 1.5 litres should be taken daily. Lie down on a hard bed. The foot of the bed must be four inches higher than the head, buttocks should be higher than the rest of body in order to facilitate the introduction of the liquid through the rectum. The vessel containing hot water for the enema should be suspended at a height of three feet from the body. The nozzle should be introduced in the rectum to allow the water to go in. Let the water go into the rectum, retain it for two to three minutes before going to the toilet. Enema

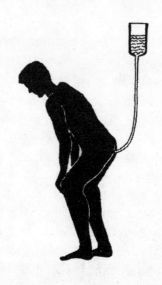

therapy helps when constipation is very severe and benefits women in leucorrhoea (white discharge)

Water Therapy

Several chronic diseases have been found cured by a simple method called water therapy. According to Japanese Sickness Association several diseases such as headache, hypertension, obesity, arthritis, rheumatism, sinusitis, rhinitis, bronchitis, asthma, hyperacidity, constipation, irregular menstruation are cured by water therapy. In this therapy 5 glasses of water (1.26 Kg) should be taken early in the morning. Do not take any hot beverage or a soft drink for next 45 minutes after drinking water. Some may have loose stools. But in a short period everything comes back to normal and symptoms of relief from the disease will be seen. Experiments have shown that hypertension takes one month, diabetes two weeks, gastritis one week and constipation one or two days to be cured.

Suncharged Water (white charged water)

It can be prepared by exposing water to direct sunrays for 4 to 6 hours. For colour charged water, specific prescribed colour bottles are used. Drink about 1 litre (4 glasses) charged water in the morning. Nothing should be taken within one hour of taking this water. Start with two glasses of water and gradually increase the amount to four glasses. This therapy cures acute as well as chronic diseases such as headache, blood pressure, anaemia, gout, paralysis, acidity, cough, asthma, tuberculosis, meningitis, liver disorders, brain troubles, gastritis, dysentry, constipation, piles, diabetes, irregular menstruation, leucorrhoea (white discharge), cancer of uterus, ear, nose and throat disorders. According to the Japanese Sickness Association, cancer can be cured within six months, tuberculosis and diabetes within one month, hypertension within 3 to 4 weeks, constipation and gastric trouble within ten days with this treatment. Store white charged water a day before its use in a copper container or earthern pot. Drink water before sunrise. Avoid eating oil, spices, chillies, condiments etc. Avoid this therapy in case of diseases like dropsy, jaundice, ascites, rheumatism, rheumatic fever etc.

Rejuvenation Therapies

Siddha vaidya, *shirodhara*, *nasaya*, *rasayana*, *siddha* massage, *panchkarma*, sandalwood treatment, *abyanga* and acupressure are various rejuvenating therapies that trigger changes in mind and organs of the body to bring balance and harmony to the overall system which helps to increase beauty and retain youth.

Shirodhara is a thin thread of warmed oil which is poured over the forehead and scalp that calms the mind, pacifies *vatha*, cleanses, calms and balances the nervous system, relieves stress and improves the body's beauty.

Shirodhara is usually repeated three to four times a week for optimal benefit.

Nasaya is a procedure aimed at reducing waste products from the head, throat and nose in human body. It is used in headaches, sinusitis, nervousness, migrains, stiff neck, running eyes, ear infections, hearing loss, loss of smell and many more ailments which ultimately affect health and beauty.

Rasayanas is a beneficial treatment for the face and scalp encompassing a head to toe routine along with other treatments such as massage (*abhyanga*), steam (*svedana*), use of herbs, pastes and mask (*snehana*), foot reflexology, aromatherapy, colour therapy, crystals and gems. These body treatments leave your skin looking and feeling fresh and healthy.

Siddha massage promotes relaxation, calming of *vatha*, *kapha* and *pitha*. It balances and increases the circulation to the body's largest eliminative organ—the skin. It increases—lymph flow, strengthens the immune system and relieves muscle tension. *Siddha* massage helps to increase the production of collagen and elastic fibres and aids in the removal and prevention of wrinkles by increasing suppleness of the skin.

Abyanga is recommended for muscle soreness, joint pain, nervousness, tension, stress, lack of energy, fatigue and tiredness, paralysis, poor digestion, poor elimination, sleeplessness all of which are necessary to enhance the beauty of the skin and body.

Sandalwood treatment which is best suited for the skin, has been used for centuries in meditation and medicine. It is a disinfectant and astringent, creates spiritual cleansing as well as cleansing of the physical body unlocking trapped fluids and toxins stored in the skin tissues.

Panchkarma – meaning five actions, is an ancient scientific system for detoxification. It rejuvenates the whole system, brings youthfulness and strength to the body and calm openness to the mind, cleaning and relieving waste materials in the body.

Acupressure therapy is used to treat disorders by pressing various pressure points (nearly 600 reflex points) on the skin of body.

Yoga Routine to Keep Young (30 Minutes Daily)

The regular practice of yoga asanas as in following table will be beneficial to maintain good health and youth. A sound mental health is key to good health and beauty of your body. A regular yoga practice in the morning and/ or evening provides excellent results. Start yoga session with warming up exercises. You must practice *shavasana* at the end, followed by meditation for sometime.

Table: Recommended Routine for beginners (30 min)

Warming up exercises	:	5 minutes
Surya Namaskar Asana	:	5 minutes
Padmasana	:	2 minutes
Halasana	:	3 minutes
Chakraasana	:	2 minutes
Sirshasana/Salambha Sirshasana	:	3 minutes
Natrajaasana	:	2 minutes
Yog Mudra	:	3 minutes
Shavasana	:	5 minutes

Padmasana (Lotus Posture): Keep right foot on the left thigh and the left foot on the right thigh. Keep hands on the heels, the back (spinal column) and neck erect. Padmasana is widely described as a meditative posture. The therapeutic

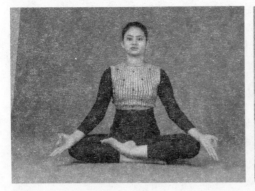
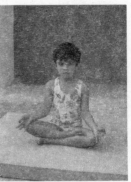

advantage of this position include developing physical and mental stability. It calms the nerves, relieves stiffness of knees and joints, supplies blood to abdominal region and the entire body is kept in complete equilibrium.

Surya Namaskar Asana: This asana involves various bending forward and backward postures and can prove to be excellent caretaker of the health if practised regularly. This asana comprises the following positions:

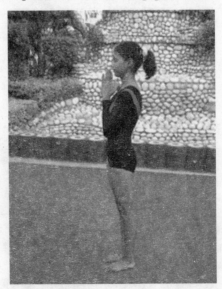

Stand erect and fold hands

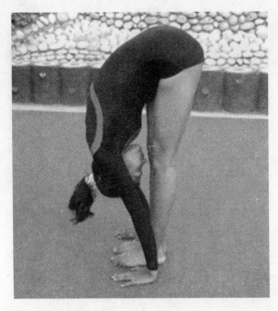

Inhale slowly. Raise both hands upward, stretched. Bend forward touching the floor with both hands.

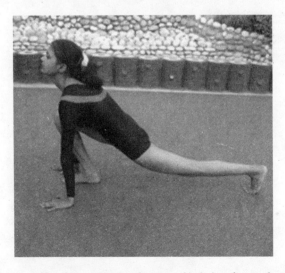

Hold breath for few seconds, then put both hands on the floor raising the head and stretching left leg backward.

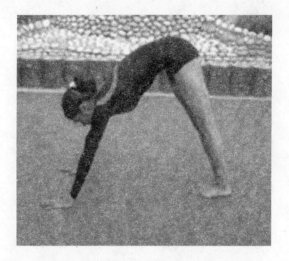

Stretch right leg too and raise the body.

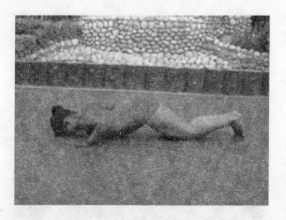

Lower the chest, touching the floor with chin.

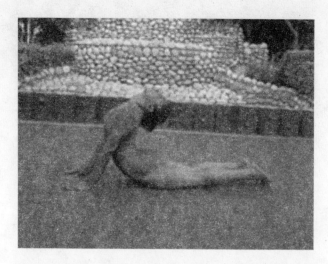

Raise head, trunk, hips, thighs and knees from floor.

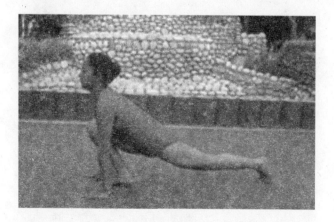

Bring right foot forward and left leg stretched back.

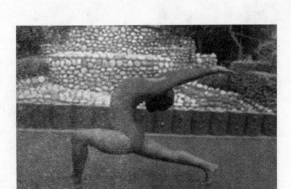

Raise the body with hands backward.

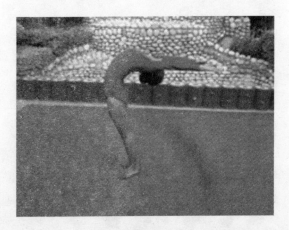

Bend backward with raised hands and feet joined.

Return to the original standing position with folded hands.

Surya namaskar asana has several benefits such as activating all the glands of endocrine system. It leaves good effect on the stomach, spine, lungs and chest. The asana invigorates the facial tissues, the central nerve system and slims all the organs of the upper part of the body.

Halasana (The Plough Posture): Lie on the back, arms stretched by the sides. Raise the legs slowly stretched vertically, then lower the legs behind the head until the tips of feet touch the ground. Remain in this position for 15-20 seconds breathing regularly, return to the standing position, relax for 15-20 seconds and repeat the posture. Do not strain if you have stiff spinal column. Halasana keeps the spine supple and healthy, helps relieve digestive problems, provides blood to the facial skin, revitalises the nerves and muscles of upper part of the body and back, has regenerating effect on the glandular system, clears menstrual disorders, prevents fat from forming on stomach, waist, hips and removes exhaustion and fatigue.

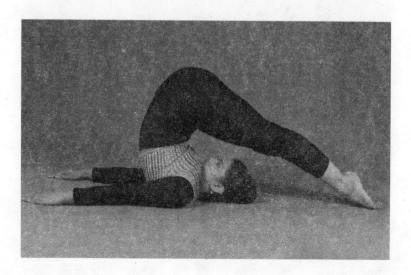

Salambha Sirshasana/Sirsh asana: Sirsh Asana (Head Stand Posture) is also called "The King of Asanas". To do this asana, kneel in front resting forearms, interlocked fingers on head. Slowly raise the knees and the hips, knees off the ground in steps. Straighten the legs perpendicular to the floor. Remain in this position for sometime, then return to initial position. In the beginning, if you are

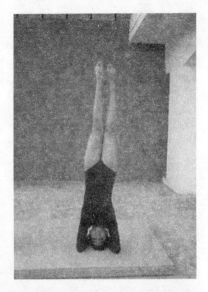

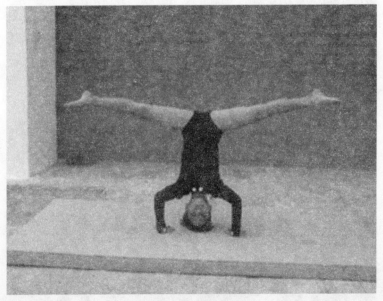

unable to practice this asana, take support of the wall. Now lift shoulders. Throw your legs backward or forward slowly. Therapeutic advantages of this asana include increased blood circulation in the head and upper portion of the body. It removes fatigue, builds up energy, improves concentration and will power, strengthens entire body, promotes growth, has beneficial effect on endocrine and digestive system and increases facial beauty.

Salambha sirshasana has therapeutic advantages similar to sirshasana. To do this asana, take position of sirshasana and bring both legs horizontal and parallel to the ground. This posture is extremely beneficial for the facial skin, scalp disorders, hair loss and disorders of genito urinary and reproductive organs.

Chakrasana (The Wheel Posture): In this posture the body is made to appear like a wheel which is a good stretching exercise to almost all the skeletal muscles. To do this asana, lie on your back. Bring your palms under the shoulders. Now raise your back and buttocks off the floor. Curve your spine resting the crown of your head on the floor.

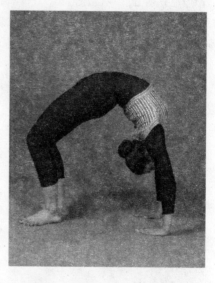

Straighten your arms and arch your spine upwards as high as possible. This is Chakrasana. This asana has various advantages. It renders the spinal column flexible and develops the thoracic cage, strengthens the muscles of the abdomen, thighs, shoulders and arms. This asana regenerates kidneys and helps to make body strong and energetic.

Natrajaasana: Natraja posture is dedicated to Lord Shiva. This posture generates vigour, vitality, potency, flexibility to the body. It strengthens the bones, enhances digestive power, leaves a good effect upon spine and improves eyesight. Perform asana as shown in the illustration and stay in this position for 8-10 seconds. Perform posture on both legs one by one.

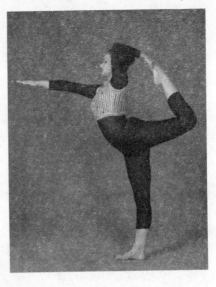

Make three rounds on each side daily.

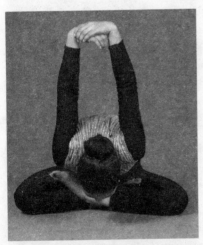

Yog Mudra (The symbol of yoga): Sit in padmasana keeping the spinal column upright. Place the hands behind the back and grab the wrist of one hand with the other. Lean forward gently without straining or jerking the spinal column. Benefits of this asana include remedy for constipation, toning up the abdominal muscles/ organs, exercising the lungs. It also helps flow of blood from the lower region to upwards, has a curative effect for asthmatics, corrects disorders of the spine, strengthens the digestive system and enhances sexual potential.

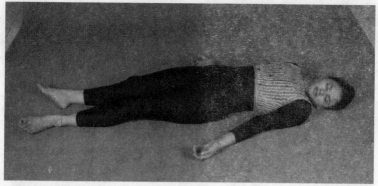

At the end of yogic routine, shavasana is performed to give mental relief.

Mudras to Fight Ageing

There are various mudras helpful for remaining young without any medication and tears. A regular practice heals many body diseases by the magic of hands.

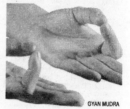

GYAN MUDRA

Gyan Mudra: Touch the tip of the thumb with the tip of the index finger, keeping the remaining fingers straight. To achieve better results practise this mudra while mediating in padmasana or vajrasana.

Vajrasana is a sitting posture in which thighs are arranged in the form of a vajra. Sit between the heels, not on them as Muslims sit for their *namaz* prayers.

Gyan mudra helps in concentration of body and mind and cures mental disorders like depression, anger, laziness, crankiness, weak memory, sleeplessness, madness and hysteria. Practise this mudra as long as possible anywhere, any time, while working, walking, sitting, lying and travelling.

Prithvi Mudra: In this mudra press the tips of ring finger and the thumb. It helps to maintain the balance in our body, removes all kinds of physical weakness, helps to gain weight (not overweight), increases the lustre of skin and makes it glow.

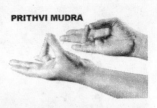
PRITHVI MUDRA

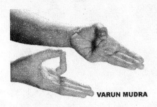
VARUN MUDRA

Varun Mudra: When the tips of thumb and the little finger are pressed together, this is varun mudra. The regular practice of this mudra removes dryness of our body and restores moisture. The deficiency of water contents in human skin leads to ageing. This mudra can be practised as and when needed.

Vayu Mudra: Keep the index finger on the base of thumb and press it with thumb. The practice of this mudra helps to decrease the level of the wind or air elements in the body which encourage ageing process in the body.

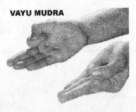
VAYU MUDRA

The benefits include curing rheumatism, arthritis, gout, stiff neck, palsy of face and cervical spondylosis.

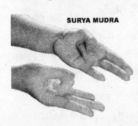
SURYA MUDRA

Surya Mudra: Bend the ring finger pressing with thumb as shown in illustration. The regular practice of this mudra 5 to 15 minutes daily in the morning and evening helps to reduce weight besides relieving mental tension—the biggest cause of ageing.

Jalodarnashak Mudra: Bend and touch the little finger at the base of thumb and press it with thumb, keeping the remaining three fingers straight. The mudra helps to decrease the water elements in the body thus enhancing glow in the skin.

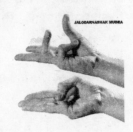
JALODARNASHAK MUDRA